Elizabeth Wo[illegible]ion as a dietitian after following the dietetics course at Leeds Polytechnic, already being a holder of a biological sciences degree from Leicester University. She has gained great expertise in helping people with food-related diseases and enjoys the challenge of devising appetizing and nutritious recipes from unusual ingredients, not least because her husband is a vegetarian and she caters for a growing family.

Virginia Alun Jones was research fellow to Dr Hunter at Addenbrooke's from 1982 until 1986. As well as contributing to this book and *The Allergy Diet*, she has presented the results of the team's work at scientific meetings in this country and Europe. She has written numerous articles for among others the *British Medical Journal*, the *Lancet*, and the *Journal of the Royal College of General Practitioners*.

John Hunter is a Consultant Physician at Addenbrooke's Hospital, Cambridge and a recognized authority on the subject of food allergy and intolerance. He developed an interest in food in relation to diseases of the gut in response to the need of the many sufferers of irritable bowel syndrome attending his out-patients' clinic. He has contributed over 60 research papers to major medical journals including the *Lancet, Nature* and the *British Medical Journal*.

POSITIVE HEALTH GUIDE

THE FOOD INTOLERANCE DIET BOOK

Delicious recipes for food allergy diets

Elizabeth Workman, SRD
Dr Virginia Alun Jones
Dr John Hunter

MARTIN DUNITZ

To Maureen Hunter,
who contributed many of the recipes in this book

First published in the United Kingdom in 1986
by Martin Dunitz Ltd, 154 Camden High Street, London NW1 0NE

British Library Cataloguing in Publication Data
Workman, Elizabeth
The food intolerance diet book.—
(Positive health guide)
1. Food allergy 2. Food allergy—
Diet therapy—Recipes
I. Title II. Alun Jones, V.
III. Hunter, John IV. Series
616.97′5 RC596

ISBN 0-948269-15-4
ISBN 0-948269-16-2 (pbk)

Phototypeset in Garamond by Book Ens, Saffron Walden, Essex
Printed by Toppan Printing Company (S) Pte Ltd, Singapore

***Front cover photograph** shows: Chicken in mango sauce (see page 88); Courgette and apple salad (see page 51)*
***Back cover photograph** shows: Melon shells filled with fruit (see page 114)*

CONTENTS

INTRODUCTION

Since we published our first book *The Allergy Diet* in 1984, interest in the possibility that various symptoms and diseases are caused by everyday foods has increased in the most astonishing way. With one in three of the population suffering from the irritable bowel syndrome and one in eight from migraine – and these are only two of the conditions we have shown to be attributed to food intolerance – it is no longer thought unusual for people to say that food, such as cow's milk or coffee, upset them and most open-minded doctors now fully accept that intolerances to food quite frequently cause problems. It is now very much easier to get assistance and understanding in dealing with this type of problem.

Some would say that too much help is available. All manner of experts, clinics and support groups have sprung up, offering advice, tests and dietary supplements. Some advocate skin tests, others hair tests, and others tell you your food allergies from a blood sample. It is hardly surprising that people get confused.

This confusion may have unfortunate effects. Whereas a few years ago many people suffered needlessly from symptoms because they did not know about the likelihood of a food intolerance causing them, we are now seeing people who believe that symptoms of any number of diseases are related to food allergy and who spend many months and often a lot of money in a fruitless search to cure the problem with a diet.

In this book we want to review the current situation with regard to medical knowledge of the causes of food intolerance, so that you can understand more clearly what is likely to help you. We describe three more conditions that can be affected by diet, in addition to the original eight we discussed in *The Allergy Diet*. We explain which tests for intolerance may be useful and which are best avoided.

Do you suffer from food intolerance?

First of all we should stress that the majority of people have no food intolerances at all. This may seem obvious, but many people worry needlessly because they are afraid that they are eating something which may be doing them hidden harm. For example, there is now great suspicion about preservatives in food. Yet these are not poisonous and present no problem to anyone with a normal digestion – indeed, their purpose is to protect against food poisoning.

If you are healthy and not suffering from any unpleasant symptoms such as headaches or diarrhoea, then you may be quite confident that you are not suffering from any food intolerances and you should go on eating a normal, full and nutritious diet. Although we have found that some people develop symptoms after eating everyday foods such as wheat, chocolate and cheese, this does not mean that these foods are in any way poisonous. The food intolerance is an individual reaction which causes trouble only to the person concerned – just because your friend is upset by, say, eating beef, there is no reason for you to avoid it too.

Allergy or intolerance?

You may be wondering why we refer to 'food intolerance' rather than 'food allergy'. This is because there are several different mechanisms by which foods may produce upsets.

An allergy is just one special sort of upset which may be produced by a food or by other substances, such as dust mites or pollen (known as allergens). Our immune system normally works by antibodies destroying bacteria or viruses entering the body. Someone with an allergy develops abnormal antibodies which react to one of these allergens, producing allergic symptoms.

When people develop antibodies against a food, the food becomes the allergen and this is a true food allergy. The antibodies meet the food in question and combine with it to trigger off cells in the body which release chemicals such as histamine. This may lead to various symptoms, for example, wheezing and a runny nose.

In the case of allergy the antibodies may be detected in the blood by a test called the RAST test (see page 15), so food allergy is a specific and detectable condition.

Intolerance is a much wider term which covers all the different ways that foods can cause things to go wrong. Many doctors used to doubt that food caused illness because people who claimed they were 'allergic' produced negative results to the usual allergy tests. They believed that these people were making up stories or imagining things, whereas in fact it was true that food was causing their symptoms, but in a completely different way.

Some foods contain chemicals which upset certain people. A good example is caffeine, which is contained in coffee. People who are susceptible to this may develop a rapid pulse rate, headaches, painful legs or indigestion after drinking coffee. They will get similar effects if they take caffeine in other forms, such as cola drinks.

Another example of chemicals in foods causing difficulty is tartrazine, the bright orange dye which is often used in squashes and sweets. This may produce urticaria or eczema, and even changes in the behaviour of young children who are unable to tolerate it. However, on the vast majority of the population it has no harmful effect at all.

Enzyme deficiencies in the body may be another cause of problems. Enzymes are chemicals which help to digest foods and people sometimes have a lack of them. In many races the enzyme which digests the lactose – the sugar in milk – disappears from the intestine as children grow into adults. People who lack this enzyme may develop diarrhoea, wind and stomach pains when they take milk.

What is the cause of food intolerance?

We have now found a possible explanation of how these chemical changes bring about food intolerance.

Recent research suggests that food that is not digested early in the intestine is broken down further on, by bacteria living in the large intestine. This enables us to get extra nutrition from our food, but it seems that some bacteria may be able to produce harmful chemicals which cause unpleasant symptoms. If these bacteria become established in the intestine, food intolerance may be the result.

An example is sorbitol, a sugar used to flavour diabetic squashes and chocolate, because it does not upset people with diabetes in the way that ordinary sugar does. When sugar is broken down in the large intestine, hydrogen is produced and can be measured on the breath. Some people with diabetes develop diarrhoea after taking drinks containing sorbitol and it has been shown that these symptoms occur at the same time as hydrogen appears on their breath. The sorbitol is being broken down in the large intestine and producing its ill effects, and the hydrogen is a by-product of the whole process. But sorbitol is not often eaten by non-diabetic people. So how are other people's digestive systems being affected?

We have recently done a large-scale study of the development of symptoms such as diarrhoea and abdominal pain caused by food intolerance (known as the irritable bowel syndrome, see page 10). We noticed that this sort of problem often came on after women had had a hysterectomy. After an operation of this sort antibiotics are often given to prevent infection while the wound is healing, and they are very effective. However, we were able to show that women who received antibiotics were more likely to develop abdominal symptoms afterwards. We found that the bacteria living in their intestine were different from those of other women who had not developed these difficulties.

We believe that some people may begin to have food intolerances after taking antibiotics. These would seem to kill off some of the bacteria in the large intestine and allow others to take their place. These bacteria may react differently during digestion and produce unpleasant chemicals which cause symptoms to develop. Of course, this is not a reason for refusing to take antibiotics if you really need them, for example, if you have bronchitis or a urinary infection. However, it is a very strong argument for taking antibiotics only when they are clearly necessary.

The conditions caused by food intolerance

It is now believed that several quite different diseases may be caused by food intolerance. A full list is given in the table opposite. We described many of these conditions in our previous book, but since that was written we have evidence that diet can affect two further conditions: Crohn's disease and hyperactivity in children. Many people are also interested in the relationship between diet and arthritis, and we discuss this on pages 12–13.

Here are brief descriptions of the conditions discussed in our original book:

Irritable bowel syndrome which is sometimes called spastic colon. The symptoms are bad abdominal pain and distension, together with diarrhoea or a very variable bowel habit. Symptoms are often developed after gastroenteritis or long courses of antibiotics. This condition is more common among women than men.

Migraine also affects more women than men and often runs in families. It is a severe headache, usually affecting only one side of the head at a time. Associated symptoms are nausea and vomiting.

Asthma has wheezing and difficulty in breathing as its main symptoms, and at night these may be accompanied by coughing.

Rhinitis is the medical name for a persistently runny or stuffed-up nose. The symptoms are similar to a common cold, but do not come and go. Rhinitis is a persistent condition.

Coeliac disease is a condition in which gluten, a protein found in wheat, rye and barley, damages the lining of the small intestine so that food is not properly absorbed, leading to a number of difficulties including diarrhoea, bone disease and failure to grow, weight loss and possible anaemia.

As these symptoms can be caused by several other conditions, it is vital that your doctor confirms the diagnosis before you start on any dietary treatment for coeliac disease.

Conditions caused by food intolerances

- Irritable bowel syndrome
- Migraine
- Asthma
- Rhinitis
- Coeliac disease
- Eczema
- Urticaria
- Cow's milk sensitive enteropathy
- Crohn's disease
- Some types of arthritis
- Hyperactivity in children

Eczema is common in both children and adults – it is an itching red rash, often on the insides of elbows and knees, which may scale and crust.

Urticaria is a very common skin condition, especially among children. Large, red, itchy blotches can appear anywhere on the body. There may also be swelling of the lips and mouth.

Cow's milk sensitive enteropathy mainly affects babies who are bottle-fed before the age of four months. The symptoms are severe stomach pain (colic), diarrhoea, eczema, vomiting and a runny nose.

Further conditions related to food intolerance

All the conditions just described have been recognized as possible causes of food intolerance for some time. We now discuss in more detail new findings on three more conditions. For these, treatment needs careful medical supervision and you should not start a diet without your doctor's agreement.

Crohn's disease

Since just before the Second World War the number of people with this disease has increased fifty times over, so that there are now about eight people in every 100,000 of the population who have Crohn's disease. It usually affects children and young adults and more women have it than men. The symptoms include diarrhoea, pain in the stomach, weight loss and anaemia. The bowel may become narrowed, leading to obstruction and the only really successful treatment until recently has been surgery, with the removal of the diseased part of the bowel. Drugs such as steroids may temporarily hold the disease in check, but they often have unpleasant side effects.

The discovery that Crohn's disease was related to diet was made entirely by accident. A young woman who came to our clinic in Cambridge was thought to have the irritable bowel syndrome and was put on the exclusion diet (see page 17). After this had been started, we received the results of tests which told us that she did, in fact, have Crohn's disease. She was called back to the clinic so we could start her on a course of steroids. When she came in, it was discovered that her condition had improved dramatically. She found her symptoms were caused by wheat and by avoiding this she has remained well ever since, with no other treatment being necessary.

Since our first discovery, we have successfully treated over 100 people with diet. Not everyone with Crohn's disease is intolerant to wheat. We find that many foods can be responsible. Cereals and dairy products are the most common and some people are intolerant of several foods. For this reason, every food must be tested separately to ensure that it does not cause trouble. Many people found to have Crohn's disease come into hospital undernourished and so we first build them up with artificial feeding, often with an elemental diet. This consists of food which has been broken down to its constituent chemicals, such as amino and fatty acids and sugars, with minerals and vitamins added. After one or two weeks on the elemental diet most people find that their symptoms clear up completely and they are then able to go on to test foods.

We are able to treat 80 per cent of people with Crohn's disease successfully by diet, but it is not suitable for all. Diet will not cure an abscess or severe narrowing of the bowel – these certainly need surgery. It is therefore very important if you have Crohn's disease not to start any diet without your doctor's agreement and encouragement. This is particularly important if you have become undernourished. Your doctor will be able to help you obtain the elemental diet. You may also need supplements to become sufficiently nourished before starting on your diet, which will require careful working out by your dietitian. We do not recommend that people with Crohn's disease try to treat themselves by following an exclusion diet without medical support. Nevertheless, anyone with Crohn's disease being treated by diet will find the information and recipes given in this book extremely useful.

Arthritis

Many people are confused about the meaning of the word arthritis. It means swelling of the joints and there are numerous forms of arthritis, which may be caused by diseases as different as damage to the nerves or bleeding into the joints. No diet can help all these conditions.

Probably the most common form, especially among women, is **osteoarthritis**, which is believed to be caused by the wear and tear of the joints, particularly in the hips and knees. This sort of arthritis will not be helped by diet, unless of course weight reduction has been recommended by your doctor, to alleviate the pressure on the joints.

Gout is caused by sharp crystals of uric acid forming in the joints. The uric acid comes from the breakdown of chemicals known as purines. Although most doctors now treat gout with drugs, which block the formation of uric acid or increase its excretion in the urine, some still recommend a diet which avoids foods rich in purines. These are found in protein-rich foods, in particular offal (liver, kidneys), peas, beans, sardines, pilchards, anchovies, herrings and fish roes. Gout was therefore one of the original forms of arthritis to be treated by diet. Treating rheumatoid arthritis by diet is not so simple.

Rheumatoid arthritis is a disease of the connective tissues, particularly affecting the tissues around joints. It causes inflammation and, eventually, stiffening of the joints concerned. This form of arthritis is more common among women than men and affects up to thirty-eight women per thousand of the population at some time in their lives.

This is the form that has caused the most interest and controversy as far as diet is concerned. Several different diets have been promoted by doctors and herbalists, but unfortunately none has proved to be entirely successful (see pages 14–16 for some examples of these). The role of diet in arthritis is far from established. Although a number of doctors have reported they have a few patients with rheumatoid arthritis who have found that foods have definitely caused their problems, a large number do seem to improve for a short time only because of the placebo effect – if they think the treatment is doing them good, it will.

However, we are now treating people with an exclusion diet specially adapted for arthritis, and we have been successful in relieving symptoms in seven out of twelve people. For full details of the diet, see pages 20–3.

Hyperactivity

Many children behave badly and it has become almost fashionable to call a child hyperactive who is simply energetic and noisy. But there is a clear distinction between **overactivity**, which is due to excessive energy and **hyperactivity**, a condition that needs special treatment.

Very few children suffer from hyperactivity. The majority who have the condition are boys aged between one and seven. They have a sustained increase in physical activity, together with poor concentration, impulsive behaviour and temper tantrums. Associated with this condition may be poor eating and sleeping habits, abnormal thirst, and learning and behavioural problems. Many also suffer from headaches, asthma, hay fever and catarrh.

The most famous findings about diet and hyperactivity were made by Dr Ben Feingold in the United States. His diet, based on the elimination of artificial colours and flavours, aspirin and natural salicylates found in some fruits and vegetables, helped 30 to 50 per cent of the children he was treating to improve. Hyperactivity is also linked to other factors such as chemicals (aerosols, disinfectants, perfume) and dust.

Many paediatricians working with hyperactive children have dismissed the Feingold diet and at present there seem to be as many arguments against treatment by diet as for it. However, a careful study at the Hospital for Sick Children, Great Ormond Street in London reported success with dietary treatment carried out on children with this problem. Of the seventy-six children treated, twenty-one recovered, forty-one improved and only fourteen showed no improvement. These children were put on a much stricter diet than Dr Feingold's. Not only additives caused trouble. Foods such as cow's milk, chocolate, wheat, oranges, cheese and eggs affected the children. Sugar, which had been blamed by many previous workers, was found to affect very few of the children.

With a child known to be hyperactive it would seem reasonable to start on the exclusion diet (see page 17). This excludes all the relevant foods and, by reintroducing the foods as instructed, you may find the solution. When dealing with children it is, of course, especially important to make sure that sufficient food, minerals and vitamins are provided, to allow for the needs of growing. For example, calcium supplements may be necessary if a suitable milk substitute is not used.

Please note that a child should undertake an exclusion diet only with the approval, and under the supervision, of a medical specialist. The final diet must always be checked by a trained dietitian.

Tests for food intolerance

As we have already shown, food may cause symptoms in different ways. Clearly no single test can be relied upon to establish whether someone has a food intolerance or to discover the foods that cause problems. There are so many tests on offer these days that you may wonder where to begin. We shall now review the various tests that are available and explain where they may be helpful.

Skin tests

These were developed by the classical allergists of the early twentieth century. An extract of a suspected food is injected into the skin, either by putting a small quantity on the skin and pricking through, or by injecting a small amount immediately beneath the skin (this is called an intradermal injection). If the test is positive, the site of the injection will swell up and be surrounded by an area of inflammation. As only one skin prick is necessary for each food, a whole battery of tests may be done at the same sitting.

This type of test may be very useful when someone suffers from a genuine food allergy, but it will not cause a reaction in anyone who is, for example, lacking the enzyme which breaks down milk sugar. So, despite the negative skin test, this person would still show symptoms after drinking milk. Skin tests may be negative in many people with food-related conditions such as migraine, diarrhoea and hyperactivity.

As most people don't know the mechanism by which their food is upsetting them, and as skin tests of this sort are by and large only available in private clinics which are expensive, they are probably not the best tests to begin with.

Tongue test

This is a modification of the skin test, but the food extract is placed under the tongue to see if it provokes a reaction. We have found it to be disappointing and unreliable.

Radioallergosorbent test (RAST)

This is a more sophisticated form of the skin test. Blood from people with genuine food allergy contains antibodies to the foods concerned and these can be detected in the laboratory by a very sophisticated analysis. Again, this test is negative in people who do not have a true allergy but who do have a food intolerance caused by a different mechanism. It has the same limited use as skin tests.

Cytotoxic test

In this test a sample of blood from the donor is mixed with food extracts. Then a few minutes later changes in the blood cells are observed under a microscope. As only a small quantity of blood and a small quantity of food extract are needed, a whole series of tests may be done on a single specimen of blood, so that the donor may be given a detailed report on possible food intolerances.

In theory this test is enormously attractive, but we have found that in practice it, too, is of little help to people with intolerances. Researchers have not yet confirmed that the blood cells of people with food intolerance react against food chemicals, although they may in people who have true allergies. Most independent scientific studies have shown this test to be unreliable, and certainly this is our experience of it. Many people come to see us claiming that they are unable to eat foods because their blood cells have reacted to samples of the foods in a cytotoxic test. Yet we find that when they really do eat them, nothing untoward happens. For example, we have given wheat to a woman who agreed to do a 'blind' test. She had been told she had a wheat intolerance, but she had no reaction at all when she was given wheat extract without knowing.

Hair tests

Many laboratories offer to diagnose your food intolerances by analysing the minerals in a specimen of your hair. Minerals such as mercury, cadmium and arsenic are deposited in your hair as it grows. It is thought that a deficiency of a mineral can explain why some people react to certain foods. The amount of minerals in your hair sometimes reflects the amount in your body at the time the hair was formed – but of course in the case of people with long hair, this may have been many months before.

The link between mineral changes and food intolerances remains to be proved, and even if you have a hair analysis done, you will still have to confirm yourself that the suspected foods cause trouble when you actually eat them. We do not recommend this technique – the main value of mineral analysis of the hair is to detect the arsenic deposited in murder victims!

Minerals in the blood

A number of minerals are detectable in the blood and mineral analysis is offered by a number of laboratories on the same principle as detecting minerals in the hair. In practice, the significance of the levels of the various chemicals is poorly understood. Zinc is known to be very important for forming various enzymes and chemicals, and yet the way it works is still largely a mystery to us. Certainly, many people who are shown to have low levels of zinc in their blood in these tests don't appear to benefit when extra zinc is provided in their diet.

Since many of the other minerals being investigated are understood even less well than zinc, we do not have much faith in this type of mineral analysis for detecting food intolerance.

Testing by diets

It is our view that because many foods produce effects by different mechanisms in different people, the only accurate way to see which foods upset you is to eat the food in question and see what happens. Whereas there have been such poor results with the other tests, our success with 70 per cent of people coming to our clinic supports our method.

We believe the essential first step if you think you may have food intolerances is to start on our exclusion diet. If this is successful the symptoms will disappear and foods can be reintroduced one by one so that you can find out exactly which are causing the symptoms.

Here we outline our exclusion diet, which we introduced in our first book. Apart from helping you detect your food intolerances, the advantage of this diet is that it is a healthy one, including fresh and wholesome foods. Arthritis sufferers who wish to try a diet should refer to page 21 for instructions on the special exclusion diet for arthritis.

People with Crohn's disease should take only an elemental diet and spring or distilled water for between ten and fourteen days. If this clears all their symptoms they should then reintroduce foods, starting with those that are allowed on the exclusion diet. Our patients have used the elemental diet known as E028, which is made by Scientific Hospital Supplies Ltd of Liverpool. It is available on prescription in the United Kingdom.

Following the exclusion diet

1. For the first two weeks keep strictly to the diet outlined in the table on page 18. It is essential to continue for the full two weeks. If you take a day off, you will have to start again from the beginning.
2. In the first fortnight it is wise to exclude any foods besides those listed in the table that you suspect may have upset you.
3. During the second week you should eat as wide a variety of the allowed foods as possible. Keep an accurate diary of every food you eat, which symptoms you have, and when. You should find you steadily improve during the second week. Any setbacks you suffer during this time will probably have been caused by one of the foods eaten in the previous twenty-four hours.
4. If your symptoms haven't improved after two weeks, it is unlikely that food intolerance is the cause of your problem. Return to normal eating and ask your doctor about other treatment.

If the symptoms disappear you can go on to find out what foods upset you in the reintroduction phase.

Rules for reintroduction

1. See the table on page 19 for the order of reintroduction.
2. Continue to keep your diary, listing foods eaten, the symptoms you have, and when. This is very important.
3. How you begin reintroducing foods depends on which condition you have. For migraine, irritable bowel syndrome, asthma, rhinitis and hyperactivity, one food should be introduced every two days. For eczema and

Foods for the Addenbrooke's exclusion diet

(for lists of foods containing prohibited ingredients, see pages 25–7)

	Not allowed	*Allowed*
Meat	preserved meats, bacon, sausages	all other meats
Fish	smoked fish, shell fish	white fish
Vegetables	potatoes, onions, sweetcorn	all other vegetables, salads, pulses, swede and parsnip
Fruit	citrus fruit, eg, oranges, grapefruit	all other fruit, eg, apples, bananas, pears*
Cereals	wheat, oats, barley, rye, corn	rice, ground rice, rice flakes, rice flour, sago, Rice Krispies, tapioca, millet, buckwheat, rice cakes
Cooking oils	corn oil, vegetable oil	sunflower oil, soya oil, olive oil, safflower oil
Dairy products	cow's milk, butter, most margarines, cow's milk yoghurt and cheese, eggs	goat's milk,† soya milk, sheep's milk, Tomor margarine, goat's and sheep's milk yoghurt and cheese, soya cheese
Beverages	tea, coffee – beans, instant and decaffeinated, fruit squashes, orange juice, grapefruit juice, alcohol, tap water (except for cooking)	herbal teas, eg, camomile, fresh fruit juices, eg, apple, pineapple, tomato juice, mineral, distilled or deionized water
Miscellaneous	chocolate, yeast, preservatives, nuts	carob, sea salt, herbs, spices In moderation: honey, sugar

* Some fruits, especially overripe ones, contain small amounts of yeast, but the quantities rarely cause any problems.

† A few people coming to our clinic have reported that goat's milk upsets them. We now therefore recommend soya milk in preference to goat's milk. However, you may find that you have no trouble with goat's milk and its products. But we do advise you to be wary of it if you have any sort of milk intolerance.

Reintroduction of foods

The order for reintroduction:

1. tap water
2. potatoes
3. cow's milk
4. yeast – take 3 brewer's yeast tablets or 2 tsp baker's yeast
5. tea
6. rye – test rye crispbread and, if yeast was negative, rye bread
7. butter
8. onions
9. eggs
10. oats – test as porridge oats
11. coffee – test coffee beans and instant coffee separately
12. chocolate – test plain chocolate
13. barley – pearl barley, added to soups and stews
14. citrus fruits
15. corn – test cornflour or corn on the cob
16. cow's cheese
17. white wine
18. shell fish
19. cow's yoghurt – test natural yoghurt, not flavoured
20. vinegar
21. wheat – test as wholemeal bread, or if yeast upsets you, test as wheat flakes.
    NB: wheat produces its effects slowly, so test for twice as long as other foods.
22. nuts
23. preservatives – fruit squashes, canned foods, monosodium glutamate, saccharin

urticaria, a period of a week may be necessary. We advise that one food is tested each day for Crohn's disease, starting from the elemental diet. You will also need to continue using the elemental diet as a supplement for a fortnight or so.

4. The time it takes for symptoms to show varies. Don't expect this always to happen immediately after you have eaten a food. Sometimes symptoms appear so slowly that they are hardly noticeable. Look back in your diary and see when you were last really well, as this will help you spot the food that has caused the trouble.
5. Eat plenty of the food that you are testing. If after the last test day you show no symptoms, you may assume that the food is safe to eat in normal quantities.
6. If a food is made up of more than one ingredient, test the ingredients before the food.

7. If you have a bad reaction, flush out your system by drinking plenty of water. Some people find that adding a little bicarbonate of soda helps.
8. At the end of reintroduction, go back and test all the foods you think have affected you to make sure that this is the case.
9. Once you have identified the foods that upset you, ask your doctor to arrange a visit to a dietitian to make sure the diet you are planning to follow is nutritionally adequate.

When testing is finished

Once you have completed the testing outlined above, you will have discovered which foods are causing your symptoms. Now you need exclude only the foods to which you are intolerant.

If you have problems with only one or two foods, this shouldn't be too difficult. As you will have probably discovered during your exclusion diet, there are very acceptable substitutes for most common foods. You have to be willing to experiment and give yourself a chance to get used to new flavours and textures. The recipes and suggestions in this book are here to help you.

However, if you find you have a long list of intolerances, you should seriously reconsider the feasibility of controlling your symptoms by diet. You should discuss this with your doctor.

People with coeliac disease must always keep to their gluten-free diet to avoid damage to the small intestine. Gluten is found in many manufactured foods as well as wheat, rye and barley. (For further information about coeliac disease, and recipes for the diet, see *The Gluten-Free Diet Book* by Dr Peter Rawcliffe and Ruth Rolph, in this series.)

Intolerances can change

It is important to remember that food intolerances can come and go. Some people discover that after excluding a food for several months they lose their intolerance. For this reason it is worth reintroducing the foods you are avoiding every six months or so, to see whether they still cause symptoms.

Unfortunately, it is also possible that in the future you may develop new intolerances. Operations, courses of antibiotics, virus infections and gastroenteritis attacks can all be reasons for this. It may be obvious to you which food has caused your symptoms, or you may have to go through the testing process all over again to discover new intolerances.

Arthritis: testing by diet

As we mentioned earlier, many different diets have been claimed to relieve rheumatoid arthritis. They are often based on diets eaten in countries where arthritis is rare. Unfortunately, most of these have been found to be disappointing.

Dr Dong's diet was devised in the 1940s and is based on a typical diet from China, where arthritis is relatively unknown. It is rich in fish and excludes red meat, fruits, egg yolk, dairy produce, additives, spices and chocolate. Although many people have claimed that the diet has helped them, a controlled trial failed to reveal any differences between those who followed Dong and those who ate an ordinary diet.

We believe this diet, although nutritionally adequate, excludes too many foods for it to be followed happily for a long time, and it lacks the flexibility of the exclusion diet – there is no point in avoiding a food unless you are quite sure that eating it causes trouble.

The Eskimo diet As a lot of fish is eaten by Eskimos and they hardly suffer from arthritis at all, it has been suggested that enriching the diet with the polyunsaturated fatty acids found in fish might help arthritis sufferers. However, a recent study reported in the *Lancet* showed that the benefit was limited. The treatment group had less morning stiffness and fewer tender joints after twelve weeks on this diet, but when they stopped it they appeared to deteriorate more quickly than the other group who received the average American diet. Besides, the relief experienced during the diet was far from complete. In our view there is little point in following a restrictive diet if it does not give total benefit.

The acid-reducing diet is based on the idea that acids produced in the body during digestion cause arthritis. It is true that uric acid is formed in gout and avoiding foods that contribute to this is recommended (see page 13). Otherwise, there is little proof to back this theory.

The acid-reducing diet differs from Dr Dong's in that it encourages dairy products and avoids fish, tea and coffee. Apart from this it is very similar and lacks scientific support.

The exclusion diet for arthritis

We are confident that people with arthritis who wish to try a simple dietary approach will come to little harm if they follow the diet laid out in the table on page 22 for three weeks. Once you have adhered to this diet for three weeks, you can go on to the reintroduction and testing of foods. The order in which you should test foods is shown in the table on page 23. Each food should be tested for four days. If your symptoms do not return after this time, you can assume the food is safe and go on to try another food. (For instructions on following an exclusion diet and reintroducing foods, see pages 17–20.)

Foods for the exclusion diet for arthritis

(Foods eaten should be fresh or frozen. Canned food and packet foods should be avoided if they contain food additives.)

	Not allowed	*Allowed*
Meat	red meats, (eg, lamb, beef, pork), bacon, preserved meats, sausages	chicken, rabbit, turkey
Fish	smoked fish, shell fish	white fish
Vegetables	onions, tomatoes	all other vegetables, potatoes, salad, pulses, beans, lentils, peas
Fruit	citrus fruit, (eg, oranges, grapefruit)	all other fruit (eg, apples, bananas, pears)*
Cereals	wheat, rye, oats, barley, corn, rice, ground rice	tapioca, sago, millet, buckwheat
Cooking oils	corn oil, vegetable oil	sunflower oil, safflower oil, soya oil, olive oil
Dairy products	cow's milk, butter, most margarines, cow's milk yoghurt and cheese, eggs	soya milk, Tomor margarine, goat's milk products (eg, yoghurt and cheese),† sheep's milk products
Beverages	tea, coffee – beans, instant and decaffeinated, fruit squashes, orange juice, grapfruit juice, tomato juice, tap water (except for cooking), alcohol	herbal teas, fresh fruit juices (eg, apple, pineapple), mineral, distilled or deionized water

* Some fruits, especially overripe ones, contain small amounts of yeast, but the quantities rarely cause any problems.

† A few people find goat's milk upsets them, so now we recommend soya milk in preference to goat's milk. However, you may find that you have no trouble with goat's milk products. But we do advise you to be wary of it if you have any sort of milk intolerance.

	Not allowed	*Allowed*
Miscellaneous	sugar, chocolate, yeast, Marmite, yeast extract, nuts, coloured toothpaste, preservatives	salt, herbs, pepper, spices – in moderation, white toothpaste, bicarbonate of soda, cream of tartar

Reintroduction of foods for arthritis

The order for reintroduction:

1. milk
2. tea
3. tap water
4. lamb
5. rice
6. butter
7. onions
8. beef
9. eggs
10. yeast – take 3 brewer's yeast tablets or 2 tsp baker's yeast in water
11. rye – test rye crispbread first then, if yeast was negative, test rye bread
12. coffee – test coffee beans and instant coffee
13. pork
14. wheat – test as wholemeal bread
15. chocolate
16. citrus fruit
17. tomatoes
18. cheese
19. corn – test cornflour or corn on the cob
20. white wine
21. shell fish
22. sugar
23. oats
24. yoghurt
25. nuts
26. preservatives – eg, fruit squashes, canned foods with food additives, sausages, smoked fish, saccharin, etc.

It is very important for anyone following the diet for rheumatoid arthritis not to stop any pills that have been prescribed until it is quite clear that the diet has relieved the symptoms. If you do stop them too early you may suffer considerable pain. Again, we would emphasize that it is essential you have your doctor's agreement before starting a trial to discover whether your arthritis can be helped by diet.

Advice on following a restricted diet

The purpose of this section is to help you when shopping for a restricted diet. We'll show you which foods not to buy, but also how many foods are available to you.

Always check the label

You already know which foods not to eat from your exclusion diet tables, but some of these are contained in manufactured products where you may not expect to find them. It is therefore extremely important always to check the lists of ingredients on the labels of any products you may buy to ensure that they don't contain any forbidden items.

The table opposite gives some guidelines on products which are most likely to contain certain prohibited ingredients, and so the labels on these products must be carefully checked. There is a more comprehensive list in *The Allergy Diet*. When you are checking labels for forbidden foods, check also for additives. These are often listed under their E numbers (see the appendix, page 120). Further information on additives can be obtained from the leaflet *Look at the Label*, published by the Ministry of Agriculture, Fisheries and Food, and the British Food Manufacturing Industries Research Association publication, *Food Additives*. On the exclusion diet it is wise to try to avoid additives as far as possible but, as this can sometimes be difficult, on page 123 we list additives which rarely produce symptoms. Foods containing these additives may be included on an exclusion diet with relatively little risk of you having any problems.

If you are in doubt about any ingredients listed on a food label, the best policy is not to include that food on the exclusion diet. Look out for labels which state that the product is additive-free – there are plenty of these around nowadays.

But what is there left to eat?

When you are first confronted with the exclusion diet it looks as if it would be almost impossible to follow, because so many familiar foods are not allowed. The recipes here show how you can eat an interesting and nutritious diet while you sort out your food intolerances. However, many of the recipes contain unusual ingredients, which you may think will be hard to find.

What we want to do now is to show that many of the foods used in the recipes, and that you can use in your own creative cookery, are easily available in great variety from the supermarket shelf. One of us went to the main supermarket in a small market town, and to the food section of a big chemist's shop, and systematically noted down which foods were available that could be enjoyed on the first stage of an exclusion diet, both as fresh ingredients and as prepared foods.

Foods to avoid or be wary of on a restricted diet

The following foods are likely to contain forbidden ingredients. Avoid the foods in column 1. Always check the labels of foods in column 2.

Ingredient	*Foods containing the ingredient*	*Foods likely to contain the ingredient*
*Wheat**	Bread: eg, white, wholemeal, wholewheat, granary Cakes and biscuits	Beverages: cocoa, drinking chocolate, 'bedtime' drinks Rye bread, crispbreads
	Fish: cooked in batter, breadcrumbs, batter or sauce Flours and cereals: ordinary wheat flours, bran, wheatgerm, semolina, pasta, noodles	Cheese: spread, processed Fish: canned, paste
	Meat: pies, sausage rolls	Fruit: pie fillings Meat: canned, ready meals, pâté, sausages, paste
	Pastry Puddings: packet puddings	Puddings: ice cream, mousses, custard powder
	Soups: canned and packets	Vegetables: canned in sauce, instant potato powder
	Miscellaneous: stuffings, packet seasonings, pepper compounds	Miscellaneous: spreads (sweet and savoury), curry powder, gravy powder, stock cubes, baking powder, bottled sauces, sweets
Yeast	Bread: except soda bread Any products containing bread	

* Products with any of the following listed on the label are likely to contain wheat: wheat starch, edible starch, cereal filler, cereal binder, cereal protein.

Ingredient	*Foods containing the ingredient*	*Foods likely to contain the ingredient*
Yeast (Cont'd)		
	Buns made with yeast, eg, teacakes, crumpets Dairy products: cheese, buttermilk, soured cream, yoghurt, synthetic cream Fermented beverages: eg, wine, beer Fruit juices (commercial) Grapes, sultanas, currants, plums, dates and prunes, overripe fruit Malted milk drinks Meat products containing bread, eg, sausages, meat loaf, beefburgers Vinegar and pickled foods Bottled sauces	
	Yeast extract	Vitamin products: most B vitamin products contain yeast
Corn†	Bleached white flour Cornflakes Cornflour Custard powder Gravy browning	Baking: mixtures for cakes and biscuits, baking powder Bottled sauces Cakes and biscuits
	Margarine, vegetable oil and salad dressings containing corn oil Sweets sweetened with corn syrup	Ice creams Instant puddings Jams, jellies and spreads Tortillas
Cow's milk and cow's milk products‡	Malted milk drinks Junket Custard Milk chocolate	Biscuits Bread, bread mixes Breakfast cereals Cakes, cake mixes Gravy mixes

† Products with any of the following listed on the label are likely to contain corn: corn starch, oil, syrup, cornmeal, edible starch, food starch, maize oil, glucose syrup, vegetable oil, dextrose.

‡ Products with any of the following listed on the label contain cow's milk: milk, butter, margarine, cream, cheese, yoghurt, skimmed milk powder, non-fat milk solids, caseinates, whey, lactalbumin, lactose.

Ingredient	*Foods containing the ingredient*	*Foods likely to contain the ingredient*
		Puddings, pudding mixes Ice creams Ready meals Sauces Soups Sausages Sweets, eg, fudge, toffee Vegetables canned in sauce
Eggs (yolk, white or lecithin)	Cakes Pastry Batter Egg noodles and pasta Lemon curd Mayonnaise	Biscuits Malted milk drinks Puddings and mixes Soups

Obviously the availability of foods will vary from place to place and at different times of the year – it was spring when we compiled this list. What we hope our list will do is convince you that you will be able to find food you will enjoy in your local shops. Following an exclusion diet doesn't have to be expensive either.

Canned foods A few people report reacting to a certain food when they have used it in its canned form, but not when it has been fresh or frozen, so we have been reluctant to use canned food in the recipes. However, the Food Preservation Institute say they can offer no explanation for this, and point out how strict the laws about food preparation, preservation, labelling and sale are. We have therefore extended the list of useful foods available from the supermarket and chemist in order to encourage you to test canned foods, and to use them to make following your diet easier.

Shopping for a restricted diet

We found the foods listed on the following pages, which are all suitable for use on an exclusion diet, in the supermarket in our local market town. A few of these are not suitable for people on the exclusion diet for arthritis (eg, red meat). If you suffer from arthritis, check foods listed here against the table of allowed foods on page 22.

Foods marked with an asterisk We found these were free from forbidden ingredients and additives, but when doing your own shopping you must always check the labels on these products.

From the supermarket

Vegetables and fruit

Fresh vegetables

Artichokes, globe
Asparagus
Aubergines
Avocados
Beansprouts
Beetroot
Cabbages
Calabrese
Carrots
Cabbages
Cauliflowers
Celeriac
Celery
Chicory
Chillies
Chinese leaves
Courgettes
Cress
Cucumber
Garlic
Ginger root
Greens
Horseradish
Leeks
Lettuce
Mushrooms
Okra
Parsnips
Peas, mangetout
Peppers:
  green
  red
  yellow
Radishes
Salsify
Swede
Sweet potatoes
Tomatoes
Vine leaves
Watercress

Frozen vegetables

Beans:
  broad
  green
Broccoli
Brussels sprouts
Carrots
Mushrooms
Peas:
  garden
  mangetout
  petit pois
Peppers:
  chopped
  mixed
Spinach
Mixtures:
Cauliflower florets with peas and carrots
Peas and baby carrots

Canned vegetables*

In water:
Bamboo shoots
In water and salt:
Asparagus
Beans, haricot
Carrots:
  baby
  sliced
  whole
Celery hearts
Macédoine of vegetables
Spinach, chopped
In water, salt and sugar:
Baby carrots and petit pois
Chickpeas (also called garbanzos)
Petit pois
In salt and sugar:
Passata (sieved Italian tomatoes)
In their own juice:
Tomatoes

Tomato purée

Fresh fruit

Apples:
- Bramleys
- Cox's orange pippin
- Golden delicious
- Granny Smith's
- Jonagold
- Sparta

Apricots
Bananas
Coconuts
Dates
Grapes:
- Alphonese Lavellee
- Italia
- Thompson seedless
- Waltham Cross

Kiwi fruit
Mangoes
Melons
Passion fruit
Paw paw
Pears:
- Bon chretien
- Conference

Pineapples
Plums:
- Songold

Rhubarb

Frozen fruit

Raspberries
Strawberries

Canned fruit*

In water and sugar:
Apricot halves
Black cherries
Pear quarters
In syrup:
Figs
Golden plums
Kiwi fruit
Lychees
Peaches
Pineapple
In apple juice:
Apple slices
Peach slices
Pear quarters
In apple and apricot juice:
Apricot halves
In natural juice:
Pineapple

Apple sauce

Fish

Fresh fish

Cod
Coley
Dover soles
Halibut
Herring
Herring roes
Huss
Lemon sole
Mackerel
Monk fish
Mullet
Plaice
Salmon
Sardines
Skate wings
Sprats
Squid
Trout
Whitebait

Frozen fish

Cod fillets
Coley steaks
Haddock fillets
Plaice fillets
Trout, whole

Canned fish*

In salt and water:
Pilchards
Salmon:
- Pink
- Sockeye red

Skipjack tuna
In tomato juice:
Pilchards

Meat and poultry

Fresh

Chicken (whole and portions)
Fancy continental butchery
Ground beef, lamb, pork and veal (check this is 100 per cent meat)
Joints of beef, lamb and pork
Pigeon (whole)
Poussin (whole)
Turkey (whole and portions)

Frozen

Beef (sirloin steak, diced braising steak, tripe, liver, heart)
Beefburgers 100 per cent (see note)
Chicken (quarters, thighs, drumsticks, wings, whole birds, livers)
Duckling (whole)
Goose (whole)
Lamb (liver, kidney, heart, tongues, brains, joints)
Pheasant (whole)
Pork (chops, diced, liver, kidney, heart)
Rabbit (diced)
Turkey (fillets, whole birds, livers)

Note: Some fast-food chains serve 100 per cent beefburgers, so ask!

General products

Drinks
Camomile tea bags
In bottles:* red and white grape juices, fizzy apple juice, colouring-free blackcurrant drink, colouring-free orange and lemon squashes, soda water (soda water and sodium bicarbonate)
In cartons:* apple juice, pineapple juice, red grape juice, tomato juice
Several varieties of both still and sparkling spring waters
In cans:* tomato juice, vegetable juice

Dry ingredients
Fruit:* currants (in food grade white mineral oil), dates in glucose, raisins
Desiccated coconut
A large variety of sugars
Seed pearl tapioca

Herbs, spices and seasonings
Herbs: chervil, coriander, dill, kuchai, lemon grass, green peppercorns, root ginger, sage, thyme, fresh bouquet garni
A great variety of dried herbs
Spices: a large selection of spices, including black pepper, cardamom, cinnamon, cloves, saffron and turmeric
Salts: table salt, coarse sea salt, fine sea salt

Margarines Milk-free margarine (Tomor)

Milk Dried goat's milk, soya milk

Nibbles Sunflower seeds*

Oils Olive oil, safflower oil, soya bean oil, sunflower oil

Oriental foods Brinjal pickle,* creamed coconut,* wheat-free curry powder, Indian poppadums (wheat-free), Madras spice poppadums (wheat-free), mango chutney,* wheat-free roghan josh spice blend, wheat-free tandoori curry spice blend

Preserves and honeys
Bottled in syrup:* blackcurrants, damsons, greengages, stem ginger
Cranberry sauce*
Jams containing only sugar, fruit and pectin (always check labels): apricot, blackcurrant, morello cherry, plum, raspberry, strawberry
Honeys: in great variety, including Chinese acacia, English, Mexican, mixed, Tasmanian
Sauerkraut (white cabbage and salt)
Tomato purée*

Pulses Butterbeans, haricot beans, lentils, marrowfat peas, split peas

Rices Basmati rice, boil-in-the-bag rice, brown rice, easy-cook American rice, flaked rice, ground rice, Italian risotto rice, Indian pilau rice,* long-grain rice, pudding rice

Now to move on to the foods we found at a large chemist/drug store. The varieties of the foods we found were all suitable for use by people following restricted diets but, as with the items from the supermarket, do check the labels on foods marked with an asterisk to ensure they don't contain any forbidden ingredients or additives.

From the chemist/drug store

Canned vegetables and fruit

Vegetables*

In water and salt:
Asparagus
Carrots
Celery hearts
Green beans
Peas
Spinach
In water, salt and calcium chloride:
Red kidney beans

Fruit*
In syrup:
Apricot halves
Lychees
Peach slices
Pear halves
In water and sugar:
Mango slices
In water:
Water chestnuts

General products

Drinks
Fruit juices:* pure apple juice (still and carbonated), pure pineapple juice, pure tomato juice. Apple juice in small cartons with straws, crushed apple drink in small cartons with straws
Tea bags:* peppermint, rosehip, lemon verbena, mint
Waters: a variety of sparkling spring waters
Made-up soya milk, suitable for babies

Dry ingredients
Fruits: peaches, pears
Rice: basmati, long-grain, pilau
A large variety of sugars
Gelatine:* wheat-free gelatine sachets
Arrowroot (wheat-free) cream of tartar (wheat-free)

Herbs, spices and seasonings
A selection of dried herbs
A selection of spices and Chinese curry powder (wheat-free)
Chinese five spice powder (wheat-free)
Curry pastes: hot and mild
Salts: table salt and various low-sodium salts

Nibbles Sesame crunch bars*

Oils Grapeseed, olive, sesame, soya, sunflower

Preserves and honeys
In bottles:* blackcurrants, gooseberries, black cherries
Honeys: acacia blossom, meadow flower, pure clear sunflower, pure set honey

Pulses Aduki beans, blackeye beans, mung beans, split red lentils, yellow split peas

Miscellaneous
Anchovy fillets in olive oil and salt
Diabetic mint imperials* (contain sorbitol, see page 9)
Pizza olives, bottled in water and lactic acid only
Poppadums
Soya bran
Tofu (soybean curd)

We hope that, together with the recipes, the lists will show you that the meals you eat while you're discovering your food intolerances (and, of course, after you've found the foods that cause your symptoms) can be creative, varied and delicious.

Cooking: ingredients and measurements

Opposite is a list of basic ingredients for cooking on exclusion diet. They are available from health food shops, if not from general stores. More detail on their use is given in *The Allergy Diet*. In addition to these we have found:

Carob sweets Carob coated sweets are a good substitute for chocolate bars. There are many types available, eg, carob-coated rice cakes and Kalibu coated fruit bars. However, the carob coating on most of these does contain milk so read the label carefully if you are following the exclusion or milk-free diets.

Grains and flours

Arrowroot
Buckwheat
Carob flour
Chestnut flour
Gram flour
Millet
Potato flour
Rice (brown is preferable to white)
Rice flour, rice flakes and ground rice
Sago flour
Tapioca

Dairy products
Cheese, ewe's or goat's
Milk, soya, ewe's or goat's (but see the note on goat's milk, page 18)

Commercially produced soya milk doesn't have a strong flavour and it can be used in cooking as an alternative to cow's milk. Some brands contain cane sugar sea salt and sunflower oil to enhance the flavour. You can make your own soya milk from soya flour:

Soya milk

Makes approximately 900 ml/1½ pints

150 g/5 oz soya flour
Vanilla pod, honey or concentrated apple juice (optional)

Mix flour with 1 l/2 pints water in a saucepan. Bring slowly to the boil, stirring all the time. (Caution! This mixture quickly froths over like cow's milk when boiling.) Reduce the heat and simmer for 20 minutes, stirring frequently.

The milk can be flavoured with honey, apple juice or vanilla pod. Add apple juice when the milk has cooled, otherwise it curdles.

Use as a milk substitute. Store in a refrigerator as it ferments when exposed to heat.

Savoury flavourings
Miso (wheat-free, made from rice)
Tahini (sesame spread)

Egg replacers We have not used these in the recipes as they are not suitable for use with the exclusion diet; but people following an egg-free diet alone may find them useful. **Bipro** is a pure protein powder produced from the whey in milk. It should not be used if you are on a milk-free diet. **Ener-G Egg Replacer** is made from arrowroot flour, potato starch, tapioca flour, modified vegetable gums and cereal-free leavening.

Gluten-free products These are also available from chemists and in the UK can be bought on prescription by people with coeliac disease. There is a range of breads, biscuits and pastas available. They can be made from wheat-starch, ie, wheat with the gluten removed or from a number of different flours, eg, maize, potato, rice, soya flours. Always check the ingredients to make sure they are suitable for you. We would not recommend that you use the varieties containing wheat starch if you are on a wheat-free diet.

Milk-free margarines There are several varieties eg, Tomor, Vitasieg, Vitaquell, Vitazell and Granose. These are made from vegetable oils and contain no animal fats. Some, eg, Vitaquell contain wheat germ oil and should not be used by people following the exclusion or wheat-free diets.

Soya products There are many soya desserts, such as rice puddings, custards and soya ice cream. Always read the ingredients to check they are safe for you to use.

Tofu is curdled soybean milk, or soy curd. It is very versatile and can be used in a number of sweet and savoury dishes. You will find a number of recipes using tofu in this book. It is also very nutritious, being a good source of protein.

Wheat-free tamari This is also made from soya beans and is a useful flavouring in savoury dishes. It can be used on the exclusion diet.

Cooking grains

Brown rice Wash and drain the rice. Allow twice the volume of cooking water to rice. Bring the water to the boil, add rice and salt (½ to 1 tsp). Reduce heat, cover and simmer without stirring for about 40 minutes until the rice is tender and water absorbed. Fluff rice with a fork when ready.

Buckwheat Put the buckwheat into twice its volume of cold salted water and bring to the boil. Simmer without stirring for about 15 minutes until the grain is soft and the water absorbed.

Millet Cook as for buckwheat. To enhance the flavour in some savoury dishes, millet can be dry roasted in the pan first.

A note on cans, containers and saucepans

There is no evidence that any of these affect people with food intolerances. It has been said for a long time that aluminium saucepans are dangerous because the metal tends to come off with use. However this, and the suspicion about using plastic containers for the refrigerator are environmental concerns rather than a factor in food intolerance.

In our experience, it is perfectly safe for you to use all your usual cooking utensils and containers when following the exclusion diet and afterwards.

The recipes

All the recipes in this book are as far as possible free from artificial colourings, flavourings and preservatives. They are also free from gluten (wheat, rye and barley), other wheat, corn, oats and cow's milk. If you simply want to exclude one or more of these from your diet you may choose any recipe you wish. If you are following the first stage of the exclusion diet or are excluding eggs you should select only those appropriately marked. If other foods are to be excluded you will need to examine the list of ingredients in each recipe carefully to see whether it is suitable for your diet.

Where you are advised to use a milk substitute, use any that is suitable for you, such as goat's, sheep's or soya milk.

Symbols

The symbols used in this book for the special diets are:

[★] exclusion

[W] wheat-free

[M] milk-free

[E] egg-free

[A] arthritis

Measurements

The measurements are given in both metric and imperial units. Use one system only; do not combine them.

When spoonfuls are referred to, level spoons are meant unless otherwise stated.

1 tsp (teaspoon) = 5 ml
1 tbsp (tablespoon) = 15 ml

To ensure success, check the size of the spoons you are using. Australian users should remember that as their tablespoon has been converted to 20 ml, and is therefore larger than the tablespoon measurements used in the recipes in this book, they should use 3 x 5 ml tsp where instructed to use 1 x 15 ml tbsp.

BREAKFASTS

Bertie Wooster's breakfast

Serves 2 ★ W M E A

225 g/8 oz turkey livers
seasoned gram flour for coating
120 g/4 oz mushrooms
sunflower oil for frying

Thaw the turkey livers if using frozen ones.

Chop the livers into bite-size pieces and cut out any fibrous tissues. Lightly coat with the seasoned gram flour. Wash the mushrooms, but don't peel them. If they are large, cut into slices. Heat a small amount of sunflower oil in a pan and fry the turkey livers for about 5 minutes, turning frequently. Add the mushrooms and fry for a further 5 minutes.

Serve with gram flour pancakes (see page 65) or buckwheat pancakes.

The Earl of Emsworth's breakfast

Serves 2 ★ W M E

6 lamb's kidneys
freshly ground black pepper
knob of Tomor margarine
4 tomatoes

Split the kidneys almost in half so they open to a bow tie shape. Snip out the tubing in the middle with scissors. Score the inside surface and rub in a little pepper. Dot with Tomor and place on the grill pan. Halve the tomatoes and arrange them around the kidneys. Cook under the hot grill for about 8 minutes, turning the kidneys once.

Serve with gram flour pancakes (see page 65) or buckwheat pancakes.

Jeeves's breakfast

Serves 2 ★ W M E

2 large or 4 small plaice fillets
knob of Tomor margarine
4 tomatoes
generous pinch basil
generous pinch sugar
seasoning

Place the fish fillets skin side down on the grill pan and dot with Tomor. Halve the tomatoes through their equators (they are prettier that way), place them on the grill pan and sprinkle with the basil, sugar and seasoning. Grill under a moderate heat until the fish is firm and has turned opaque all over, but be careful not to allow it to go dry.

Basil complements both tomatoes and fish.

Aunt Agatha's vegetarian kedgeree

Serves 1 ★ W M E

1–2 tbsp sunflower oil
1 small dessert apple, cored and sliced into rings
1 small banana, cut into discs
75 g/2½ oz cold cooked brown rice
seasoning

Heat half the oil in a small frying pan. Fry the apple rings for a couple of minutes on each side, then add the banana discs and fry for a further 2 minutes. Add the rice to the pan and stir well, adding further oil if necessary. Season to taste.

Serve when the rice has warmed through – the banana will have softened and almost disappeared, but the apple rings will still be intact.

BEVERAGES

Redbush tea with fresh mint

Serves 2–4 ★ W M E A

1 Redbush tea bag
2 sprigs fresh mint
600 ml/1 pint boiling water

Put the tea bag and mint sprigs into a tea pot. Pour on the boiling water and leave to brew for 5 minutes. Stir and serve.

Note: This refreshing tea is also good served chilled.

Ginger tea

Serves 4 ★ W M E

5 cm/2 in piece fresh ginger root
2½ tbsp runny honey
4 cloves
900 ml/1½ pints water

Peel the ginger and chop it coarsely. Place it in a pan with the honey, cloves and water. Bring to the boil, cover, turn the heat down low and simmer for 25 minutes. Remove the lid and simmer for another 15 minutes. Strain and serve the tea hot or cold.

This makes an excellent drink for a sore throat.

Note: If you prefer weaker tea, use less ginger.

Rice tea

Makes 900 ml/1½ pints ★ W M E

2 tbsp uncooked white rice
900 ml/1½ pints boiling water

Place the rice in a heavy-bottomed frying pan and heat gently. Stir the grains until they turn dark brown. Now tip the grains into a small pan and add the boiling water. Simmer for 1 minute. Strain and serve.

If you wish you can sweeten the tea with some honey – about 1 tsp per cup.

Peanut milk

Serves 4 W M E

600 ml/1 pint water
120 g/4 oz shelled peanuts
honey to taste (about 2 tsp)

Place all ingredients in an electric blender, and blend until a smooth milk is formed.

You can vary the flavour by substituting different nuts (almonds, cashews, etc.) for the peanuts.

Carob and banana milk

Serves 4 ★ W M E

500 ml/18 fl oz soya milk
2 tsp runny honey or molasses
2 tbsp carob flour
1 banana, peeled and sliced

Place all the ingredients in an electric blender. Blend until well mixed. Serve chilled.

Tomato cocktail

Serves 6 ★ W M E

750 ml/1¼ pints tomato juice
150 g/5 oz goat's yoghurt
120 ml/4 fl oz apple juice
mint leaves to garnish

Place the tomato juice, yoghurt and apple juice in an electric blender. Blend well. Chill well. Serve garnished with mint leaves.

Tasty tomato juice

Serves 4–6 ★ W M E

600 ml/1 pint tomato juice
1 large sprig parsley
¼ tsp marjoram
½ tsp basil
2 tsp brown rice miso

Place all the ingredients together in an electric blender. Blend until well mixed. Serve chilled.

FIRST COURSES AND SOUPS

Avocado dip

W M E

Serves 4–6

For the dip:
1 clove garlic, crushed
juice and zest of 1 lemon
2 tomatoes, skinned, seeded and chopped
seasoning
2 ripe avocados
90 ml/3 fl oz olive oil

For the crudités:
4 carrots, sliced into long strips
4 sticks celery, sliced into long strips
½ cucumber, sliced into long strips
1 green pepper, cored, seeded and sliced into long strips
1 red pepper, cored, seeded and sliced into long strips
½ small cauliflower, broken into florets

Place the garlic, lemon juice and zest, tomatoes and seasoning into a liquidizer. Blend well. Stone and peel the avocados. Add the flesh to the liquidizer and blend again. Gradually blend in the oil – add a little of the oil, blend, add a little more, blend again (as if you were making mayonnaise). Continue in this way until the mixture is creamy and pale green.

Pour the dip into a bowl. Place the bowl in the middle of a large serving dish and arrange the crudités around it.

Aubergine purée

Serves 4

W M E

2 large aubergines
1 clove garlic, crushed (optional)
2 tsp lemon juice
2 tbsp sunflower oil
seasoning
parsley, finely chopped, black olives and lemon wedges to garnish

Place the aubergines under a hot grill, turning occasionally, until the skins are black and blistering (about 15–25 minutes). Peel off the skins – do this under running cold water as the aubergines will be hot! Remove as much juice as possible by placing the aubergines in a sieve and pressing down hard with a wooden spoon or a plate.

Curried apple and carrot soup (*above and centre*, see page 48); Aubergine purée (below)

OVERLEAF: Antipodean salad (*top left*, see page 52); Marinated fried tofu (*below left*, see page 55); Mushrooms with coriander (*centre*, see page 54); Aubergine and buckwheat pasta (*right*, see page 57)

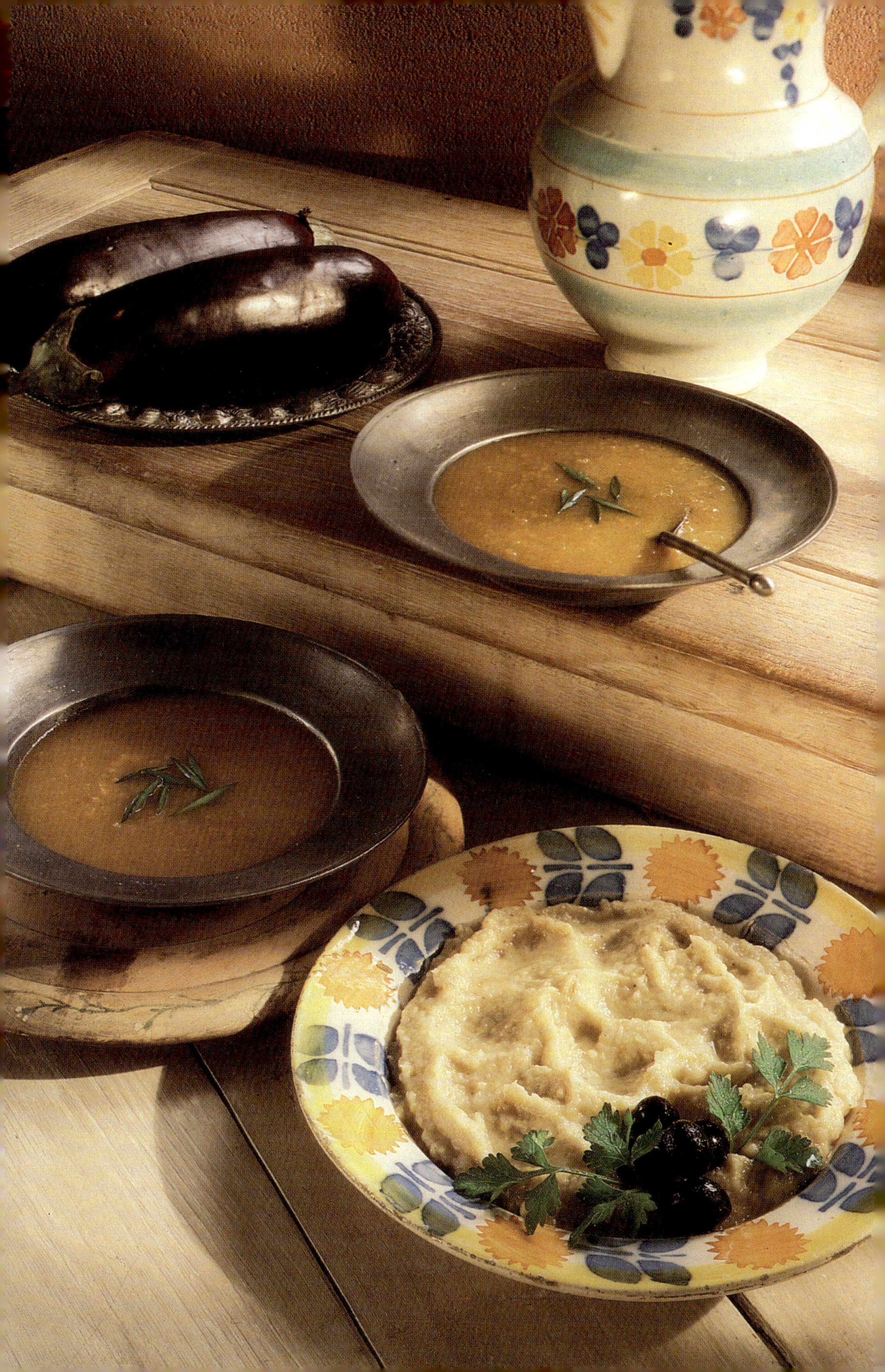

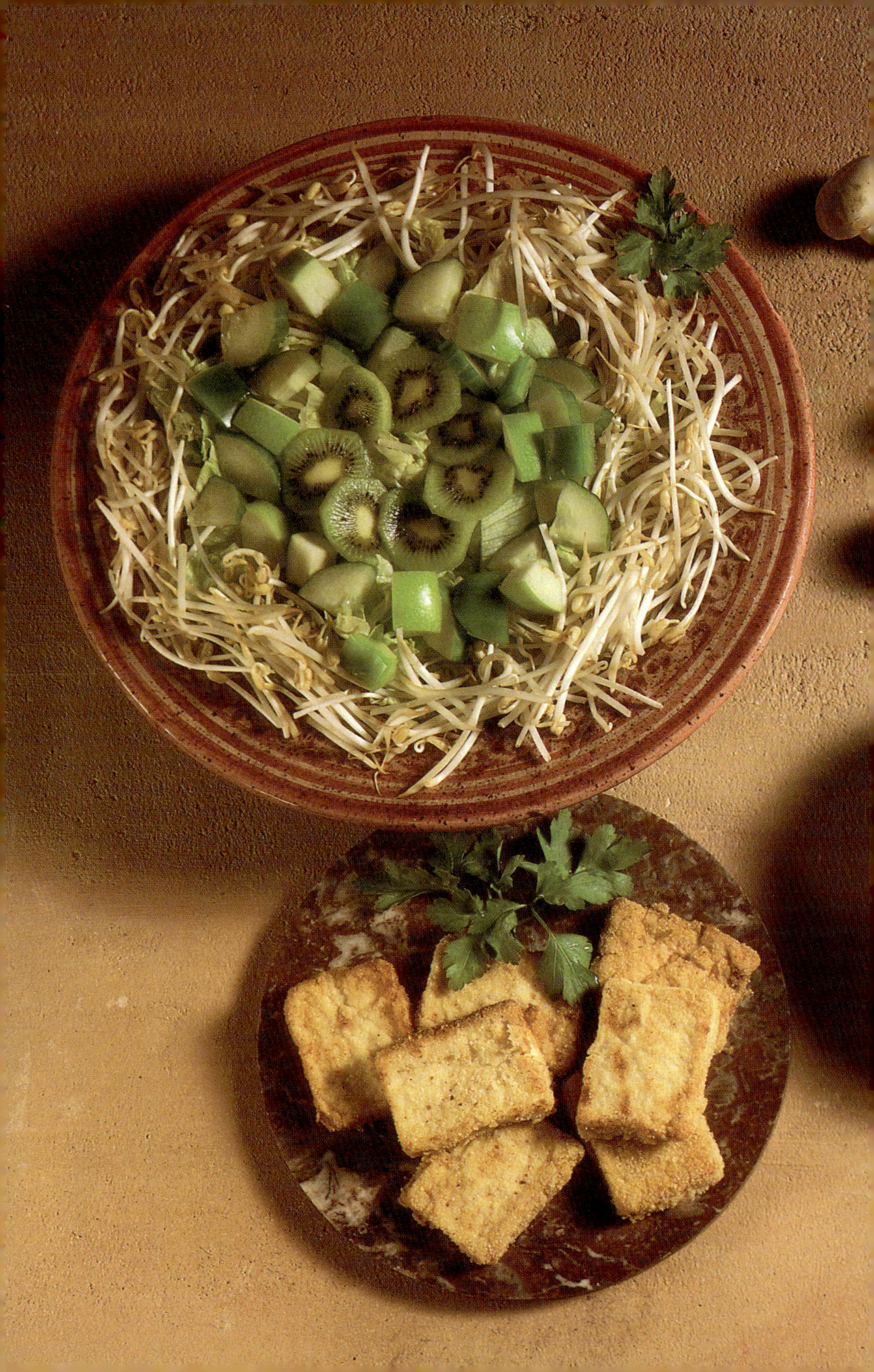

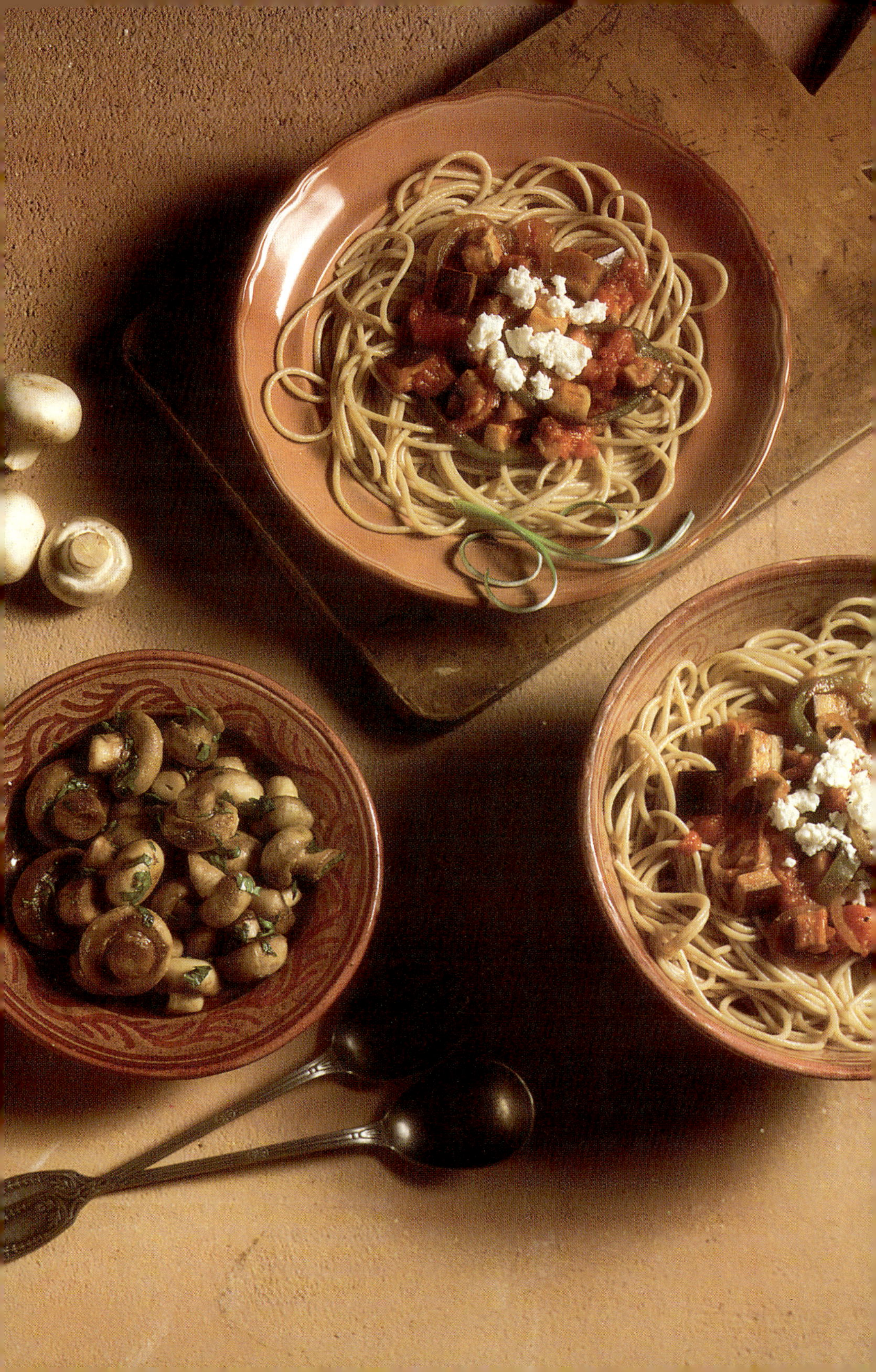

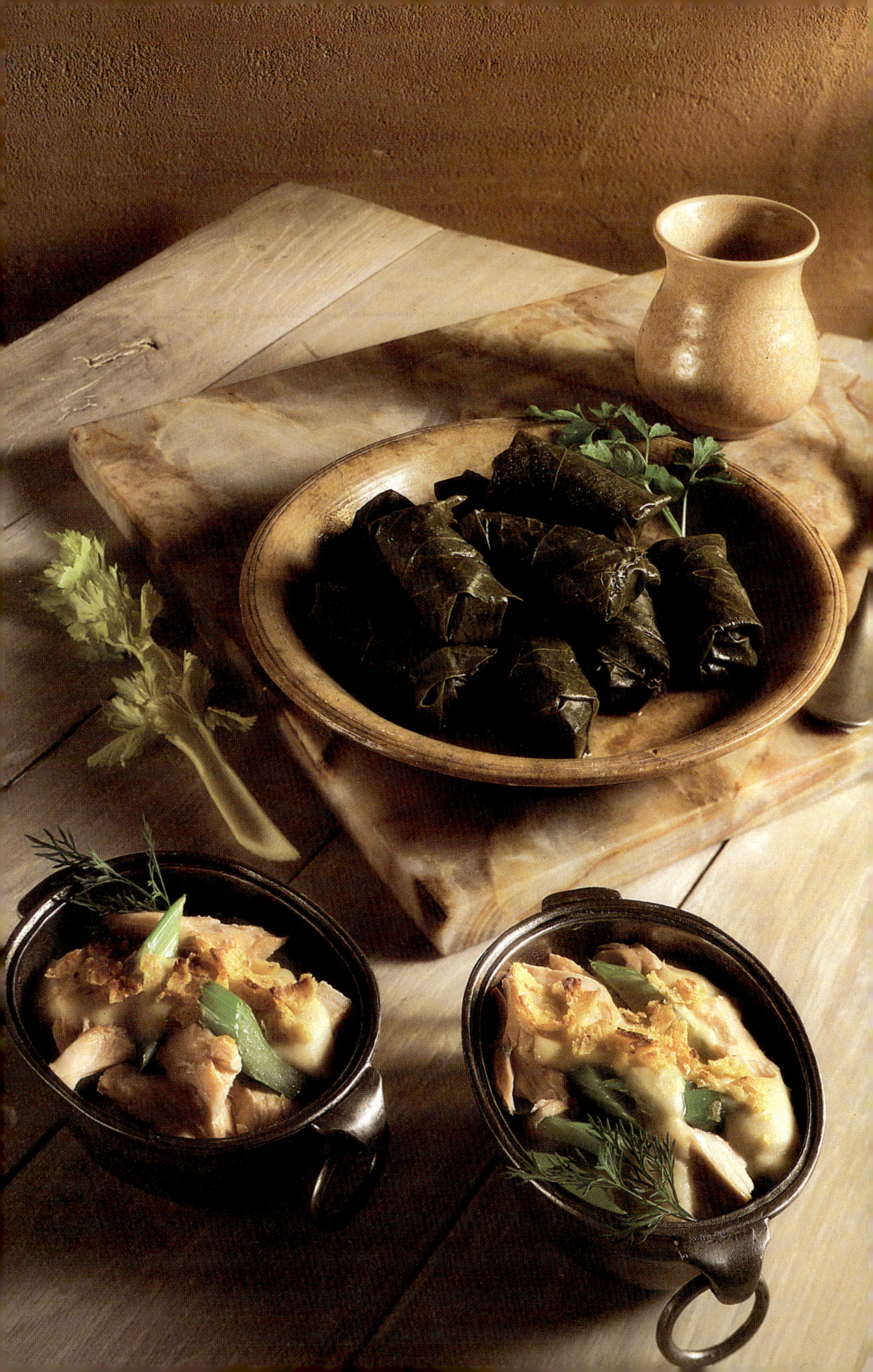

Put the aubergine flesh into a liquidizer. Add the garlic (if using) and the lemon juice. Blend, adding the oil a teaspoon at a time. The resulting mixture should be smooth and creamy. Season to taste. Garnish with chopped parsley, black olives and lemon wedges.

Dolmades

Serves 6 as a starter
Serves 3 as a main meal

★ W M E

12 vine leaves (or Savoy cabbage leaves)
225 g/8 oz minced veal or beef
1 clove garlic, crushed
60 g/2 oz cooked rice
½ tsp chopped mint
1 tsp chopped parsley
1 pinch cinnamon
1 tbsp olive oil
seasoning
a little water

Preheat the oven to 190°C/375°F/gas 5.

Blanch the vine leaves in boiling water for 2 minutes. (If using cabbage leaves, blanch for 5 minutes.) Drain carefully and leave to cool, draped round the sides of a colander.

Place the minced meat in a bowl, add the rice, herbs, spice and garlic. Mix well, Pour in the olive oil and mix to bind the ingredients. Season.

Spread out the leaves. Divide the meat into 12 portions and place each portion in the middle of a leaf. Wrap the leaves around the meat mixture. Carefully transfer the parcels to a shallow ovenproof dish. Pour a little water into the bottom of the dish and cover with a tightly fitting lid.

Place the dish in the oven and bake for 1 hour.

Note: A delicious variation is to use leftover pheasant and chopped apricots instead of the veal or beef.

Mary's salmon starter

★ W M E A

Serves 6

225 g/8 oz fresh salmon
5 black peppercorns
4 sticks celery, sliced
30 g/1 oz Tomor margarine

For the sauce:
20 g/½ oz Tomor margarine
20 g/½ oz soya flour
90 ml/3 fl oz milk substitute
seasoning

1 packet soya crisps

Preheat the oven to 200°C/400°F/gas 6.

Poach the salmon in a little water with the black peppercorns

Dolmades (*above*); Mary's salmon starter (*below*)

for 10 minutes. Fry the celery in the margarine very gently for 3–4 minutes. Flake the cooked salmon into bite-size pieces. Place the salmon in a shallow ovenproof dish and put the celery on top.

Now make the sauce. Melt the Tomor over a low heat. Add the flour and stir well. Let the mixture cook for 2 minutes. Warm the milk substitute and gradually add it to the Tomor and flour, stirring all the time. Once the mixture has come to the boil, let it simmer for 2 minutes. Season.

Pour the white sauce over the salmon and celery. Crumble the soya crisps on top and bake in the oven for 10–15 minutes.

Serve piping hot.

Turkey liver pâté

Makes 225 g/8 oz [★] [W] [M] [E] [A]

225 g/8 oz turkey livers, chopped
1 stick celery, finely chopped
120 g/4 oz Tomor margarine
1 large clove garlic, crushed
½ tsp mixed herbs
seasoning

Fry the livers and celery together in 30 g/1 oz of the Tomor for 3 minutes. Add the garlic, herbs and seasoning and cook for a further 15 minutes, stirring occasionally. Melt the rest of the margarine in a pan over a low heat.

Place the liver mixture in the liquidizer, together with the melted margarine and liquidize. Put the pâté in a bowl and cover it with foil. Chill in the fridge. Remove from the refrigerator 30 minutes before serving, to allow the pâté to soften.

Chicken liver salad

Serves 4 as a starter
Serves 2 as a main meal [★] [W] [M] [E]

120 g/4 oz haricot or butter beans
sufficient water to soak the beans
225 g/8 oz chicken livers
1 tbsp olive oil
2 sticks celery, finely chopped
2 small tomatoes, skinned, seeded and sliced

For the dressing:
2 tbsp olive oil
1 tbsp apple juice
2 tsp wheat-free tamari sauce
black pepper to taste

toasted sesame seed to garnish

Soak the beans overnight in enough water to cover. Drain. Boil in fresh water for 1½ hours. Leave to cool.

Slice the livers into thin strips. Heat the oil in a pan and fry the liver gently for a few minutes. Remove from the pan and drain on absorbent paper. Leave to cool.

Drain the beans and place them in a large serving bowl. Add the celery, tomatoes and cooled liver.

Make the dressing by combining all the ingredients. Pour over the salad and toss well. Chill. Before serving, toss once more and garnish with the sesame seeds.

Curried parsnip soup

Serves 6–8

W M E

4 medium parsnips
85 g/3 oz Tomor margarine
120 g/4 oz onion, chopped
1 clove garlic, crushed
3 tbsp rice flour
2 tsp wheat-free curry powder
1.8 l/3 pints hot beef stock (see page 90)
seasoning

Peel and slice the parsnips. Melt the Tomor in a heavy pan and add the parsnips, onion and garlic. Cover the pan and cook slowly for 10 minutes, taking care that the vegetables do not go brown. Add the rice flour and the curry powder, stirring them in to take up the fat. Gradually pour in the beef stock. Bring to the boil and simmer until the parsnips are cooked (about 20 minutes).

Liquidize the soup. Return to the pan and season to taste. Reheat and serve.

Thick celery soup

Serves 2

★ W M E A

150 g/5 oz celery
150 ml/¼ pint soya milk
300 ml/½ pint water
50 g/1½ oz orange lentils
1 clove garlic, crushed
seasoning

Wash and coarsely chop the celery. Place in a pan with the milk, water, lentils and garlic. Bring to the boil then simmer until the ingredients are soft enough to liquidize (about 5–10 minutes). Liquidize and return soup to the pan. Reheat, adding seasoning to taste.

Spinach and tomato soup

Serves 4

★ W M E

250 g/9 oz fresh spinach or leafbeet leaves and stems
4 tomatoes
300 ml/½ pint home-made jellied stock (tongue stock, see page 78)
300 ml/½ pint soya milk (or soya milk and water mixed)
2 tsp tomato purée
freshly ground black pepper

→

Wash and roughly chop the spinach or leafbeet. Chop the tomatoes. Place spinach and tomatoes in a pan with the stock and soya milk or soya milk/water. Bring the mixture to the boil and simmer until all the ingredients are heated through. Liquidize thoroughly. Return to the pan and add the tomato purée and the pepper. Reheat and serve.

Salsify and apple soup

Serves 2 ★ W M E A

200 g/7 oz salsify
1 dessert apple
20 g/½ oz yellow split peas (don't presoak)
300 ml/½ pint water
150 ml/¼ pint soya milk
seasoning
watercress to garnish

Scrape the salsify and cut into convenient lengths. Quarter the apple and remove the core. Leave the skin on to increase the fibre content of the soup. Place the salsify, apple and split peas in a pan. Add the water and bring to the boil. Lower the heat and simmer gently, covered, until the salsify and peas are soft enough to be liquidized (about 30–40 minutes).

Liquidize the mixture. Return the soup to the pan, add the soya milk, season to taste and reheat until nearly boiling. Serve, garnished with watercress.

Curried apple and carrot soup

See photograph, page 41

Serves 2–3 ★ W M E

170–200 g/6–7 oz carrots
1 dessert apple (about 50 g/1½ oz in weight)
1 tbsp soya oil
1 tsp wheat-free curry powder
15 g/½ oz brown rice miso
600 ml/1 pint very hot, but not boiling, water
seasoning
finely chopped chives to garnish

Scrub the carrots and chop them into discs. Quarter and core the apple, leaving the skin on to increase the fibre content of the soup. Heat the oil in a pan and add the carrots and apple. Sweat them in their own juices over a low heat for 30 minutes, shaking the pan occasionally and taking care that they don't burn. Next, stir in the curry powder and cook the mixture for a couple more minutes.

Mix the miso with the hot water and add this to the mixture in the pan. Liquidize. Return the soup to the pan, season to taste and reheat. Do not allow to boil or the miso will curdle.

Serve garnished with chopped chives.

Cream of artichoke soup

Serves 2–3 ★ W M E A

250 g/9 oz Jerusalem artichokes
50 g/1½ oz yellow split peas
600 ml/1 pint water
seasoning
paprika and parsley to garnish

Peel the artichokes. Don't presoak the peas, simply place them in a pan with the artichokes and the water and bring to the boil. Skim off the foam, turn down the heat and simmer, covered, for about 30–40 minutes until the split peas are soft enough to be liquidized, by which time the artichokes should be cooked.

Liquidize the mixture and season to taste. Serve good and hot, garnished with a pinch of paprika and a sprig of parsley on each bowl.

SALADS

Bean salad

★ W M E

Serves 6

120 g/4 oz red kidney beans
sufficient water to soak the kidney beans
120 g/4 oz butter beans
sufficient water to soak the butter beans
120 g/4 oz French beans

For the dressing:
2 tbsp apple juice
2 tbsp olive oil
1 pinch caster sugar
seasoning

2 tbsp chopped parsley
1 tbsp chopped chives

Soak the dried beans separately overnight. Drain. Kidney beans need to be boiled quickly in fresh water for 10 minutes, to drive off the toxins, then simmer for 1½ hours. Simmer butter beans separately in fresh water for 1½ hours.

Prepare the French beans by chopping them in 2.5 cm/1 in pieces. Boil for 10 minutes.

Meanwhile, make the dressing by mixing all the ingredients together and beating vigorously to obtain an emulsion.

While they are still warm, place all the beans in a large bowl and add the dressing, tossing well. Chill.

Stir in the chopped parsley and chives just before serving.

Bean and pepper salad

Serves 6 ★ W M E A

170 g/6 oz blackeyed beans

For the dressing:
6 tbsp olive oil
2 tbsp apple juice
1 pinch wheat-free dry mustard
freshly ground black pepper

1 medium red pepper, seeded and sliced into thin strips
1 yellow or green pepper, seeded and sliced into thin strips
1 tbsp finely chopped parsley

Place the beans in a pan with plenty of lightly salted water. Bring to the boil and simmer for 45 minutes.

Meanwhile, mix together the olive oil, apple juice, mustard and black pepper.

Drain the beans and toss in the dressing while still warm. Chill.

Just before serving, add the peppers and parsley to the beans. Toss once more to ensure that the beans and peppers are well coated with the dressing.

Carrot salad

Serves 4 W M E

60 g/2 oz sultanas
juice of 1 lemon
450 g/1 lb carrots

Soak the sultanas in the lemon juice overnight.

Finely grate the carrots and mix with the lemon-soaked sultanas. Serve with a salad dressing. Oil and lemon juice goes well with this dish.

Carrot and beetroot salad

Serves 2 ★ W M E A

2 medium young carrots
2 tbsp desiccated coconut
1 tbsp sultanas
2–3 small cooked beetroots

Wash and finely grate the carrots. Place in a bowl, add the coconut and sultanas and mix well.

Slice the beetroots into discs and arrange them around the edge of a medium-size plate. Pile the carrot mixture in the middle and serve.

Courgette and apple salad

Serves 2 ★ W M E A

2 medium courgettes
1 Granny Smith apple
60 g/2 oz sultanas
small pinch mixed herbs
seasoning
4 tbsp apple juice

Cut the courgettes into sticks and steam them for 2–3 minutes. Leave to cool. Core, quarter and slice the apple, leaving the peel on. Place the cooled courgettes and the chopped apple in a bowl, add the sultanas and mix thoroughly. Sprinkle with the herbs and seasoning and pour the apple juice over the mixture. Toss well.

Leave to marinate for 15–30 minutes, tossing occasionally, then serve.

Fennel salad

Serves 2 W M E

1 large fennel bulb
2 lettuce leaves
6 olives, stoned
1 tbsp finely chopped parsley

For the dressing:
2 tbsp sunflower oil
1 tbsp wine vinegar
seasoning

Wash the fennel and trim off the stalks. Cut the bulb thinly across to make fennel rings. Shred the lettuce leaves. Place the lettuce, fennel rings, olives and parsley in a salad bowl. Add the oil, vinegar and seasoning. Toss well and serve.

Green goddess salad

Serves 6 ★ W M E A

450 g/1 lb frozen peas
12–15 small cauliflower florets
85 g/3 oz stuffed green olives
30 g/1 oz ginger, freshly grated
7 tbsp olive oil
1 tsp grated nutmeg
seasoning
2 tbsp finely chopped parsley

Place all the ingredients except for the parsley in a pan with a closely fitting lid. Bring to the boil, turn off the heat and leave with the lid on for 5–6 minutes. Cool then chill.

Fold in the parsley just before serving.

Antipodean salad

See photograph, page 42

Serves 6

★ W M E A

½ iceberg lettuce
280 g/10 oz beansprouts
1 kiwi fruit
½ crisp green apple, cored
¼ green pepper, cored and seeded
10 cm/4 in cucumber
apple juice dressing (see page 50)

Wash, dry and coarsely chop the lettuce. Arrange it in the bottom of a large shallow dish to make a bed for the other ingredients.

Wash and dry the beansprouts. If you are using a rectangular dish, halve the total quantity and put one lot across each end. If you are using a round dish, put the beansprouts all the way round the perimeter.

Carefully peel the kiwi fruit and cut into slices crossways, to show the pretty pattern. Arrange the kiwi circles in the centre of the dish.

Coarsely chop the apple, pepper and cucumber. Place these between the kiwi fruit and the beansprouts.

Chill, then serve with apple juice dressing.

Special tomato salad

Serves 4

★ W M E

4 salad tomatoes
2 pinches mixed herbs
1 tsp granulated sugar
⅛ tsp salt
⅛ tsp freshly ground black pepper

Wash the tomatoes. Holding them over the bowl you are going to serve the salad in, cut each tomato into 8 pieces, letting the juice dribble into the bowl. Place the tomato pieces in the bowl, add the herbs, sugar and seasoning and mix thoroughly.

Oriental banana salad

Serves 1

★ W M E

1 small or medium banana
1 pinch sugar
1 pinch salt
freshly ground black pepper
1 pinch ground cumin
1 pinch cayenne pepper
splash of apple juice

Unzip the banana and slice into a bowl. Add the other ingredients and toss thoroughly.

VEGETABLES

Red cabbage

Serves 6

★ W M E

1 medium red cabbage
30 g/1 oz Tomor margarine
1 tsp sugar
1 medium green apple, peeled, cored and chopped
6–8 black peppercorns
240 ml/8 fl oz apple juice
60 g/2 oz sultanas

Discard the central stalk and coarse outer leaves of the cabbage. Finely shred the rest.

Melt the Tomor in a large pan over a gentle heat. Toss the shredded cabbage in this until all the margarine has been absorbed. Add the sugar and the apple. Stir in the peppercorns. Pour in the apple juice and bring to the boil. Turn down the heat and stew the mixture gently, tightly covered, for 45 minutes.

Add the sultanas and continue cooking in the same way for a further 15 minutes.

This dish can be served hot or cold and can be reheated slowly. Delicious with pork, duck or goose.

Baked courgettes

Serves 4

★ W M E

4 small or 2 large courgettes
6–8 tomatoes
1 clove garlic
seasoning
1 pinch oregano
1 pinch basil

Preheat the oven to 190°C/375°F/gas 5.

Cut the courgettes in half lengthways and scoop out the softer flesh in the middle. Arrange the courgette boats in a shallow ovenproof dish.

Coarsely chop the tomatoes. Crush the garlic. Mix the chopped tomatoes and their juice with the garlic, seasoning and herbs. Pour this mixture into the hollows of the courgettes, letting any extra spill over into the dish.

Bake uncovered for 30 minutes.

Mushrooms with coriander

See photograph, page 42

Serves 2 ★ W M E A

20 g/½ oz Tomor margarine
225 g/8 oz mushrooms
2 tsp finely chopped coriander leaves
¼ tsp ground coriander

Melt the margarine in a pan and fry the mushrooms over a gentle heat. Add the coriander and cook for a few more minutes before serving.

Stir-fried mixed vegetables

Serves 2–3 ★ W M E A

3 tbsp oil
1 clove garlic, crushed
2.5 cm/1 in root ginger, finely chopped
seasoning
½ green pepper, cored, seeded and chopped
½ red pepper, cored, seeded and chopped
1 large carrot, thinly sliced on the diagonal
¼ cauliflower, broken into florets
120 g/4 oz beansprouts

Heat the oil in a large frying pan. Add the garlic, ginger and seasoning and stir-fry for 1 minute. Add the prepared peppers, carrot and cauliflower and stir-fry for 4 minutes. Add the beansprouts and stir-fry for a further 4 minutes.

Transfer the mixture to a warmed serving dish and serve at once.

Note: You can use many different combinations of vegetables for this dish, following the instructions above.

VEGETARIAN DISHES

Marinated fried tofu

See photograph, page 42

Serves 2–4

[★] [W] [M] [E] [A]

280 g/10 oz firm tofu
2 tbsp wheat-free tamari sauce
2 cloves garlic, crushed
millet flour for coating
sunflower oil for frying

Cut the tofu into 1.25 cm/½ in thick slices. Mix together the tamari and crushed garlic and marinate the tofu slices in this mixture for a few hours.

Remove the tofu from the marinade and coat the slices with the millet flour. Heat a little oil in a pan and shallow-fry the tofu until golden brown, turning once.

Note: This makes an excellent substitute for meat.

Chinese-style tofu

Serves 2

[★] [W] [M] [E] [A]

1 tsp arrowroot
4 tbsp water
2 tbsp sunflower oil
1 green chilli, cut into thin strips
1 sweet red pepper, cut into thin strips
¼ tsp salt
225 g/8 oz firm tofu, cut into 2.5 cm/1 in cubes
1 tbsp wheat-free tamari sauce
4 tbsp finely chopped coriander leaves

Mix the arrowroot and the water in a cup. Heat the oil in a heavy-bottomed pan, add the chilli, red pepper and seasoning. Stir-fry for 30 seconds.

Turn the heat down low and add the tofu to the pan, mixing gently. Add the tamari and the arrowroot mixture. Stir carefully until the sauce thickens. Just before serving stir in the coriander.

Serve hot with rice and salad.

Butter bean curry

Serves 4 W M E

225 g/8 oz butter beans
sufficient water to soak the beans
1 tsp cumin seeds
3 tbsp oil
1 onion, chopped
30 g/1 oz fresh ginger, chopped
2 cloves garlic, crushed
1 tsp ground cumin
1 chilli, chopped
1 tsp ground coriander
½ tsp turmeric
4 cloves
450 g/1 lb tomatoes, skinned and chopped
300 ml/½ pint water
2 tsp garam masala
seasoning

Soak the beans in the water overnight. Drain and rinse. Cook in plenty of fresh water until tender – about 20 minutes. Drain and cover.

Dry roast the cumin seeds in a heavy-bottomed pan until they turn a darker colour. Set aside.

Heat the oil in a pan and fry the onions until soft. Add the ginger and garlic and cook for 2 minutes. Add the cumin, chilli, coriander, turmeric and cloves, the tomatoes and the water and cook until the tomatoes are soft. Mix with the beans and cook for a further 15 minutes.

Just before serving, stir in the garam masala and season to taste. Serve with rice (see page 33) and walnut raita (see page 93).

Note: If you prefer a milder curry, omit the chilli.

Aubergine supper

Serves 4 ★ W M E

900 g/2 lb aubergines
salt
180 ml/6 fl oz olive oil
2 heads chicory
450 g/1 lb tomatoes, skinned, seeded and sliced
2 cloves garlic, crushed
seasoning
280 g/10 oz goat's yoghurt
120 g/4 oz fresh goat's cheese
Tomor margarine for greasing
60 g/2 oz goat's Cheddar cheese, grated

Preheat the oven to 190°C/375°F/gas 5.

Slice the aubergines lengthways. Sprinkle with salt and leave to sweat for 30 minutes. Pat dry with absorbent paper.

Heat 120 ml/4 oz of the oil in a pan and fry the aubergine slices until golden brown on both sides. Set aside.

Chop the chicory heads and stew gently in the remaining oil for 15 minutes. Add the tomatoes, garlic and seasoning. Mix well.

Combine the yoghurt with the fresh goat's cheese.

Grease an ovenproof dish with Tomor. Place one-third of the aubergines in the bottom, then one-third of the tomato mixture, then one-third of the yoghurt mixture. Continue layering in this way until all the ingredients have been used. Sprinkle the goat's Cheddar on the top.

Place in the oven and bake for 30 minutes.

Aubergine and buckwheat pasta

See photograph, page 43

W M E

Serves 2

1 aubergine
salt
3 tbsp sunflower oil
1 clove garlic, crushed
1 onion, sliced
1 tsp dried oregano
1 small green pepper, cored, seeded and sliced
225 g/8 oz tomatoes, skinned and sliced
seasoning
170 g/6 oz buckwheat pasta (available from health food stores)
60–90 g/2–3 oz feta cheese

Slice the aubergine, sprinkle with salt and leave for 30 minutes. Rinse and drain. Heat the oil in a pan and add the garlic and onion. Sauté for 5 minutes. Add the aubergine with the oregano, pepper and tomatoes. Cook for a further 15 minutes. Season to taste.

Cook the buckwheat pasta in plenty of boiling water until it is soft but not soggy. Drain and arrange on a warmed serving dish. Pour the aubergine mixture into the middle of the pasta. Crumble the feta cheese over the top.

Serve with a crisp salad.

Turmeric rice

★ W M E

Serves 6

350 g/12 oz uncooked brown rice
1 pinch salt
½ tsp powdered turmeric
1 l/1¾ pints boiling water
handful sultanas, soaked for 3–4 hours in apple juice (optional)

Measure the rice into a large pan, add the salt and the turmeric (being careful not to spill any as it has a persistent yellow stain). Pour on the boiling water and bring back up to the boil. Stir well, cover with a tight-fitting lid and simmer for about 35 minutes or until the rice is cooked. All the water should have been soaked up and the grains should be separate.

Stir in the sultanas, if required, and serve.

Stuffed peppers

Serves 3 ★ W M E

120 g/4 oz uncooked brown rice
3 green peppers
4 tomatoes
1 tbsp soya oil
seasoning
2 tbsp chopped basil

Cook the rice (see page 33), and keep warm.

Wash the peppers. With a sharp knife, cut the tops off to make lids. Carefully remove the seeds and cores from the inside of the peppers. Steam the pepper shells for 7–10 minutes, so they are cooked but still firm. Keep warm.

Coarsely chop the tomatoes. Heat the oil in a pan and fry the tomatoes, seasoning and chopped basil until soft. Tip the cooked rice into the pan and stir it into the tomato mixture. Cook for a few minutes.

Place each pepper on a warmed serving plate, spoon the rice and tomato mixture into the peppers and replace the lids. Serve at once.

Rice tabouleh

Serves 4 W M E

150 g/5 oz uncooked brown rice
1 bunch spring onions, finely chopped
1 bunch parsley, finely chopped
1 bunch mint, finely chopped
juice of 1 lemon
3 tomatoes, coarsely chopped
3 tbsp olive oil
seasoning

Cook the rice (see page 33). Drain it and leave to cool.

Place all the ingredients in a large bowl (including the cooled rice). Mix thoroughly and season to taste.

Vegetarian paella

Serves 4 W M E

2 aubergines
salt
225 g/8 oz uncooked brown rice
2 tbsp sunflower oil
2 cloves garlic, crushed
2 onions, chopped
3 bay leaves
½ red pepper, cored, seeded and sliced
½ green pepper, cored, seeded and sliced
6 tomatoes, chopped
225 g/8 oz button mushrooms
170 g/6 oz mixed nuts, chopped
juice of 1 lemon

Dice the aubergines, sprinkle them with salt and leave for 30 minutes. Drain and rinse. Cook the rice (see page 33). Drain and keep warm.

Heat the oil in a large frying pan. Add the garlic, onions and bay leaves and cook for 5 minutes. Add the aubergines, peppers, tomatoes and mushrooms. Cook for 5–10 minutes until the vegetables are tender.

Meanwhile, place the chopped nuts on the grill pan and toast them under the grill until they are lightly browned.

Add the rice, nuts and lemon juice to the mixture in the pan. Cook gently until all the ingredients are warmed through.

Serve immediately with a crisp salad.

Note: Pulses such as kidney beans or aduki beans can be substituted for the chopped nuts in this recipe.

Vegetable dahl

Serves 2 as a main course ★ W M E

100 g/3½ oz yellow split peas
sufficient water to soak the peas
300 ml/½ pint water, or brown rice miso stock
⅓ of a cauliflower
2 medium carrots
200 g/7 oz swede
½ tsp wheat-free curry powder
2 tsp garam masala
2 tsp tomato purée
2 tbsp sunflower oil
2 tomatoes, roughly chopped
120 g/4 oz fresh or frozen peas
seasoning

Soak the split peas in the water for 24 hours. Drain and rinse. Place in a pan with the 300 ml/½ pint of water or miso stock. Bring to the boil and simmer until the split peas are soft (20–30 minutes).

Meanwhile, break the cauliflower into florets. Coarsely chop the carrots. Peel and chop the swede. Steam the cauliflower, carrots and swede until half cooked. Drain, saving the cooking water.

Liquidize the cooked split peas with the liquid they were cooked in, adding the curry powder, garam masala and tomato purée. Add extra vegetable cooking water if necessary – the final consistency should be like a cream soup.

Fry the cauliflower, carrots and swede in the oil for a few minutes, then add the chopped tomatoes and frozen peas to the pan and cook for a further 2–3 minutes. Add the liquidized dahl mixture, season to taste, and cook for 5 minutes to allow the flavours to blend.

Indian millet with yellow split peas

Serves 4 ★ W M E A

85 g/3 oz yellow split peas
sufficient water to soak the peas
170 g/6 oz whole millet
1 tbsp sunflower oil
½ tsp cumin seeds
½ tsp mustard seeds
2 sticks celery, finely chopped
1 clove garlic, crushed
½ tsp ground turmeric
½ tsp ground cumin
1 tsp ground coriander
⅛ tsp cayenne pepper
450 ml/¾ pint water
chopped parsley to garnish

Soak the peas overnight in the water. Drain and rinse.

Dry roast the millet in a heavy-bottomed pan until it starts to turn a light brown colour. Heat the oil in a pan and fry the cumin seeds, mustard seeds, celery and garlic for a few minutes. Add the split peas, millet and spices. Sauté for 2 minutes. Add 450 ml/ ¾ pint water and bring to the boil. Cover, turn heat down and cook for 40 minutes, adding more boiling water if necessary to prevent the mixture from drying out.

Turn off the heat and leave the pan to sit, covered, for a further 15 minutes. Stir quickly with a fork and garnish with chopped parsley.

Serve as an accompanying dish to a main meal.

Millet-coated split pea cutlets with apple rings

Makes 12 cutlets W M

340 g/12 oz yellow split peas
sufficient water to soak the peas
450 ml/¾ pint water
1 large onion, peeled and chopped (or 1 stick celery, chopped, if onions are not allowed)
30 g/1 oz Tomor margarine
½ tsp sage
⅛ tsp ground cloves
1 egg
seasoning

To finish:
rice flour
1 egg, beaten
millet flakes for coating
sunflower oil for frying

For the apple rings:
2 medium cooking apples
30 g/1 oz Tomor margarine
2 tbsp sunflower oil

Soak the peas in the water overnight. Drain and rinse. Place in a pan with 450 ml/¾ pint water and cook until the peas are tender and all the liquid has been absorbed. It may be necessary to drain the beans and dry them out by stirring over a low heat for a couple of minutes, if they are cooked before all the water has disappeared. Fry the onion in the melted Tomor for 5 minutes. Then add the peas, sage, cloves and the egg. Mix well, mashing the peas with a spoon. Allow to cool.

Shape the mixture into 12 cutlets on a board dusted with rice flour. Dip each cutlet into the beaten egg and then evenly coat with millet flakes. Heat the oil in a pan and fry the cutlets until golden brown and cooked through. Drain on absorbent paper. Keep warm.

Make the apple rings by peeling the apples and removing the cores. Slice into thin rings. Heat the Tomor and the oil in a frying pan and fry the rings for about 2 minutes on each side until lightly browned. Drain on absorbent paper.

Serve the cutlets with an accompanying bowl of apple rings and a green salad.

Colourful lentils

Serves 4 as a main dish
Serves 6 as a side dish

[★] [W] [M] [E]

4 tbsp olive oil
3 cloves garlic, crushed
4 carrots, chopped
1 green pepper, seeded and chopped
1 red pepper, seeded and chopped
1 tsp basil
3 sticks celery, chopped
1 tbsp brown rice miso
900 ml/1½ pints hot water
675 g/1½ lb tomatoes, skinned, seeded and chopped
280 g/10 oz lentils (don't presoak)
seasoning
2 tbsp chopped parsley

Heat the oil in a pan and add the garlic, carrots, green and red peppers, basil and celery. Cook until the ingredients are soft. Mix the miso with the hot water and add this to the mixture, together with the tomatoes. Stir in the lentils. Season to taste.

Simmer for 1 hour. Serve, garnished with the chopped parsley.

Continental lentil rissoles

Serves 4

[★] [W] [M] [E] [A]

225 g/8 oz continental lentils
sufficient water to soak the lentils
300 ml/½ pint water
2 tbsp sunflower oil
1 stick celery, chopped
1 large clove garlic, crushed
1 small green pepper, cored, seeded and chopped

1 tsp turmeric
1 tsp ground coriander
1 tsp ground cumin
¼ tsp chilli powder
seasoning
rice flour for coating (use millet flour if following arthritis exclusion diet)
sunflower oil for frying

Soak the lentils in the water overnight. Drain and rinse. Put into a large pan with 300 ml/½ pint of water. Bring to the boil then simmer gently until the lentils are tender and have absorbed all the liquid – about 30–45 minutes.

Heat the oil in a pan and add the celery, garlic and green pepper. Cook for 5 minutes. Stir in the turmeric, coriander, cumin and chilli powder and cook for 2 minutes. Add the vegetable and spice mixture to the cooked lentils. Stir well and season to taste. Leave to cool.

Mould the mixture into small rissoles and coat evenly with rice or millet flour. Heat the oil in a frying pan. Fry the rissoles until they are well browned and cooked through.

Drain the rissoles on absorbent paper before serving with brown rice, tomato sauce (see page 90) or raita (see page 93) and a crisp salad.

The rissoles can also be served cold.

SNACKS

Cucumber dip

★ W M E A

See photograph, page 92

150 g/5 oz goat's yoghurt
½ large cucumber, diced
seasoning
2 tsp finely chopped mint

Place the yoghurt and diced cucumber in the blender. Liquidize. Season, then fold in the mint. Chill.

Serve with soya crisps or diced vegetables.

Cheese dip

★ W M E A

150 g/5 oz goat's yoghurt
120 g/4 oz soft goat's cheese
4 cloves garlic, crushed
½ tsp paprika or cayenne pepper

Place the yoghurt, cheese and garlic in the blender and liquidize. Chill.

Just before serving, garnish with paprika or cayenne pepper.

Tofu spread

★ W M E

Makes 340g/12 oz

See photograph, page 92

280 g/10 oz tofu
1 tbsp wheat-free tamari sauce
1 tbsp tomato purée
1 clove garlic, crushed
1 tsp chopped basil (or 1 pinch of dried basil)
⅛ tsp salt
⅛ tsp black pepper

Place all ingredients in the blender and liquidize until smooth.

Use as a spread for sandwiches or as a creamy dip for a starter.

Salad dip

[★] [W] [M] [E]

3 cloves garlic
2 sticks celery, chopped
1 green pepper, seeded and chopped
½ tsp dried basil
4 cm/2 in cucumber, peeled and diced
2 tsp olive oil
150 g/5 oz fresh goat's cheese
2 tomatoes, skinned, seeded and sliced
seasoning

Place the garlic, celery and green pepper in a pan. Add just enough water to cover the vegetables. Bring to the boil and simmer for 8 minutes. Drain off water and stir the basil into the vegetable mixture. Leave to cool.

Place the cooked vegetables in the blender with the cucumber, olive oil, goat's cheese and tomatoes. Blend until smooth. Season. Chill.

Serve with soya crisps or diced vegetables or as part of a salad.

Bean and apple dip

See photograph, page 92

[★] [W] [M] [E]

120 g/4 oz red kidney beans
sufficient water to soak the beans
1 tbsp tomato juice
1 medium cooking apple, peeled, cored and chopped
2 tbsp goat's or ewe's yoghurt
¼ tsp salt
freshly ground black pepper
chopped chives to garnish

Soak the beans in the water overnight. Drain. Boil beans quickly in fresh water for 10 minutes, to drive off the toxins, then simmer for 1½ hours. Leave to cool, then drain again.

Place the beans, tomato juice, apple, yoghurt and seasoning in the blender and liquidize until smooth.

Serve, garnished with the chives, with diced vegetables or soya crisps.

Deep fried mung beans

See photograph, page 92

Nibbles for 2

[★] [W] [M] [E] [A]

50 g/1½ oz mung beans
sufficient water to soak the beans
sunflower oil for deep frying
seasoning

Pick over the beans and put them to soak for 24 hours in plenty of water.

Wash the beans in fresh water and pat them dry with kitchen paper.

Heat the oil so that when the beans are lowered in, in a sieve, they sizzle briskly. Cook until the sizzling dies down a bit – about 90 seconds. It is best to do the beans in two batches.

Tip the beans into a basket lined with absorbent paper. Dab off excess fat, changing the paper if necessary. Season while still hot.

Eat hot or cold, instead of peanuts or crisps.

Gram flour pancake

See photograph, page 70

Serves 1

★ W M E A

30 g/1 oz gram flour
6 tbsp water
1 pinch turmeric
1 pinch salt
1 pinch cayenne pepper
1 tbsp sunflower oil

Sift the gram flour into a bowl, and gradually stir in 4 tbsp of the water, periodically pausing to beat the mixture well, breaking up any lumps which are forming. Add the rest of the water with the turmeric, salt and cayenne pepper, and beat the mixture again.

Heat the oil in a heavy-bottomed pan. Test that it is hot enough by dropping a small blob of mixture into it. Once it sizzles it is ready. Add all the mixture and swirl it round so it covers all the base of the pan. Shake gently to prevent it sticking. After 3–4 minutes, when the first side is crisp and browning, turn the pancake and cook the second side.

Serve with a savoury filling (see below and pages 36, 66).

Savoury pancake filling

See photograph, page 70

Serves 1

★ W M E

1 tbsp sunflower oil
1 apple, cored and chopped
1 stick celery, sliced
15 g/½ oz green pepper, chopped
30 g/1 oz cold deep-fried mung beans (see page 64)
1 tomato, chopped
15 g/½ oz tomato purée

Heat the oil in a small frying pan and gently cook the chopped apple, celery and green pepper until they are soft. Add the mung beans, tomato and tomato purée. Mix well. Add a little water if necessary to make some 'gravy'. Cook the mixture for a further 5 minutes.

Serve with gram flour pancakes (above) or buckwheat pancakes.

Oriental snack lunch

Serves 2 ★ W M E A

2 medium carrots
1 clove garlic, cut in half
1 tbsp soya oil
120 g/4 oz okra
120 g/4 oz button mushrooms
340 g/12 oz beansprouts
seasoning

Wash the carrots and cut them into long, thin fingers. Rub the cut clove of garlic round a non-stick frying pan, then gently heat half the oil and start frying the carrot strips. Keep the pan covered as much as possible while cooking this dish.

While the carrots are frying in the covered pan, wash the okra, cutting the stems off as close as possible to the pod, but being careful not to cut into the pod (to prevent the glutinous middle escaping during cooking). Add the prepared okra to the carrots and cook, covered, for a further 5–7 minutes.

Wash and slice the mushrooms. Wash the beansprouts. Add both to the pan with the seasoning and the rest of the oil. Stir well. Turn up the heat and fry, covered, stirring occasionally, for a further 10 minutes (total cooking time about 20 minutes).

Chick pea and tomato lunch

Serves 2 ★ W M E

100 g/3½ oz chick peas
sufficient water to soak the chick peas
1 small green pepper
2 tbsp sunflower oil
1 clove garlic, crushed
8 tomatoes, roughly chopped
2 pinches parsley
2 pinches thyme
seasoning

Soak chick peas in plenty of water for 24 hours. Drain and rinse.

Core and roughly chop the pepper. Heat the oil in a heavy-bottomed pan. Fry the pepper with the crushed garlic until the pepper is soft. Add the chopped tomatoes to the pan, then the chick peas, herbs and seasoning. Mix well and add a little water if it is necessary in order to allow the ingredients to simmer together without drying out. Cover the pan with a tight-fitting lid and cook gently for 45 minutes.

Serve with gram flour pancakes (see page 65), buckwheat pancakes or commercial urd flour poppadums.

Cheese and fruit nut loaf

See photograph, page 70

W M E

Makes 8–10 slices

170 g/6 oz goat's Cheddar cheese
85 g/3 oz feta cheese
a little soya milk
1 large dried apricot, chopped
1 tbsp chopped hazelnuts
1 tbsp sultanas
1 large prune, chopped
extra chopped nuts to decorate

Finely grate the Cheddar cheese and combine with the crumbled feta cheese. Add enough soya milk to moisten and bind.

Place half the cheese on a large sheet of foil in a shape approximately 17 × 5 cm (8 × 2 in). Sprinkle the apricot, hazelnuts, sultanas and prune over the top. Cover with the remaining cheese. Wrap the foil tightly round the loaf, forming a sausage shape. Refrigerate overnight.

Unwrap, decorate with chopped nuts and slice to serve as a snack or with drinks.

Fruit and nut snack

See photograph, page 70

W M E

120 g/4 oz unsalted peanuts
200 g/7 oz dried apricots, chopped
200 g/7 oz sultanas
85 g/3 oz sunflower seeds
85 g/3 oz shelled walnuts, chopped

Combine all the ingredients and store in an airtight tin. Good for including in packed lunches or for serving with drinks.

FISH

Trout with cucumber

Serves 4 ★ W M E A

1 cucumber, peeled and cut into 2 cm/ 1½ in pieces
4 trout, cleaned, washed and dried
30 g/1 oz millet flour, seasoned with salt and pepper
85 g/3 oz Tomor margarine
freshly ground black pepper

Boil the cucumber in a little salted water for 3–4 minutes. Drain on absorbent paper.

Roll the trout in the seasoned flour.

Heat the Tomor margarine in a frying pan until very hot. Fry the trout, turning once, for 15–20 minutes, depending on size. Remove the fish from the pan, drain on absorbent paper and keep warm. Toss the cucumber in the pan in which the trout were cooked. Cook gently for 5 minutes. Season.

Place the trout on a serving dish. Arrange the cucumber around the fish and serve at once.

Baked stuffed trout

Serves 4 W M E

4 trout, cleaned, washed and dried
1 cooking apple, peeled, cored and coarsely chopped
2 sticks celery, sliced
50 g/1½ oz shelled walnuts, chopped
1 tbsp water
50 g/1½ oz Tomor margarine
seasoning

Preheat the oven to 180°C/350°F/gas 4.

Place the apple, celery and walnuts with the water in a pan with a well-fitting lid. Simmer gently until the apple softens. Stir well.

Grease a large shallow ovenproof dish with a little of the Tomor. Pack a quarter of the stuffing mixture into each trout. Arrange the stuffed trout in the dish. Season and dot the fish with the remaining Tomor. Bake for 20 minutes. Baste frequently.

Serve immediately from the baking dish.

Fish cakes (*above*, see page 73); Baked stuffed trout (*below*)

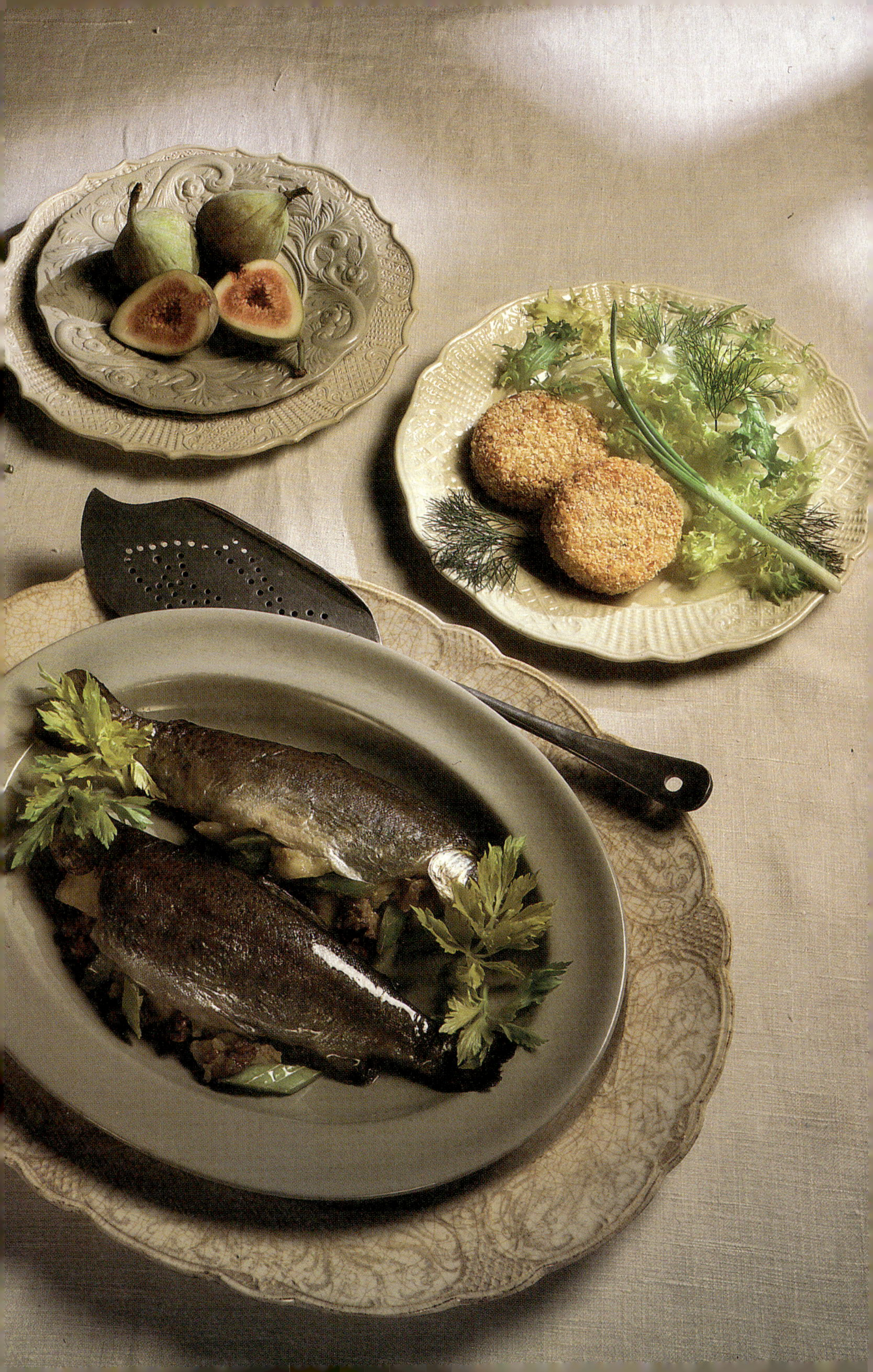

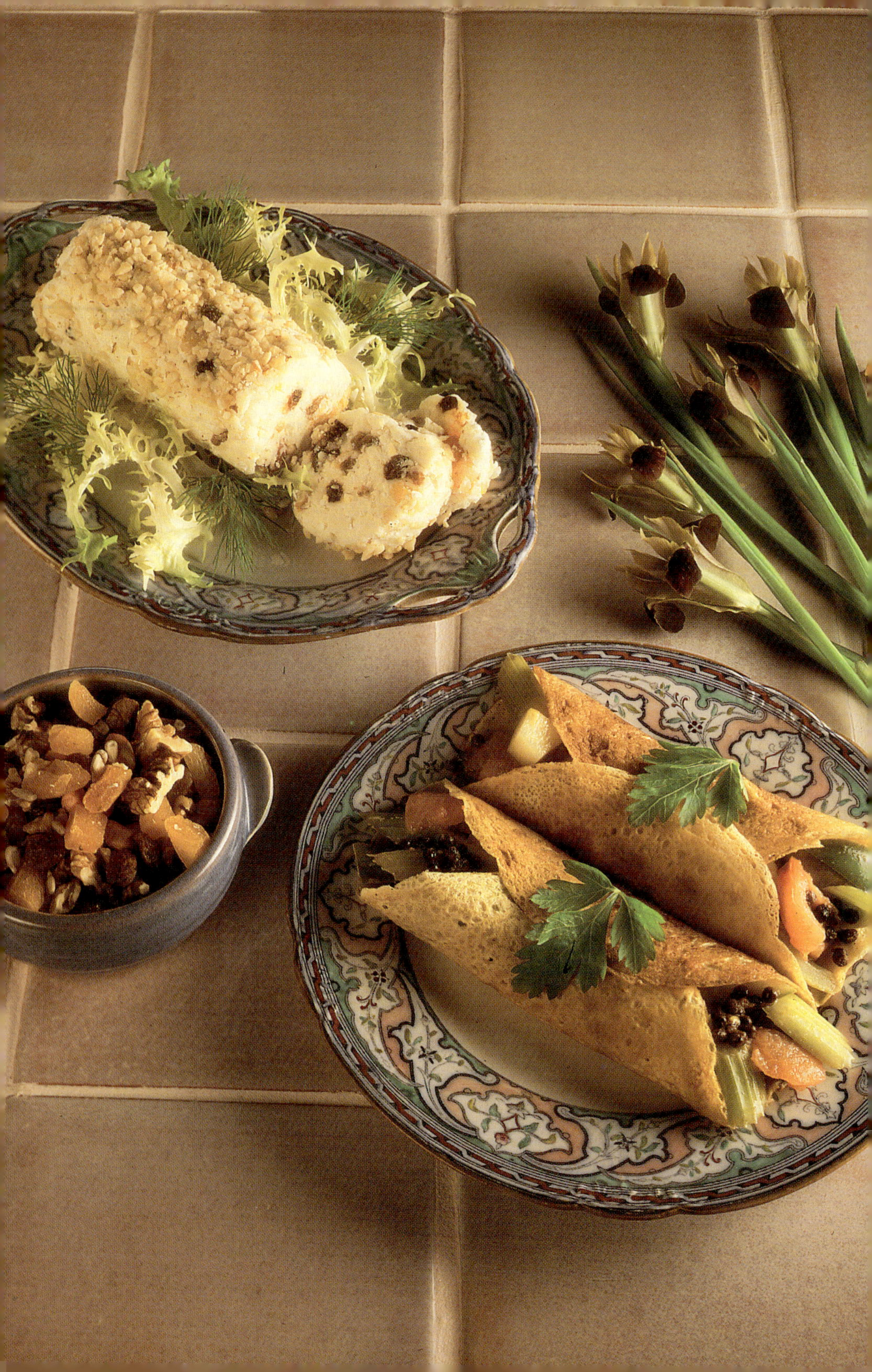

Italian halibut

Serves 4 ★ W M E

4 halibut steaks
1 tbsp olive oil
1 stick celery, finely chopped
1 red pepper, seeded and chopped
450 g/1 lb tomatoes, skinned and seeded
1 tsp basil
seasoning
chopped parsley to garnish

Preheat the oven to 200°C/400°F/gas 6.

Place the halibut in an ovenproof dish greased with a little of the olive oil. Heat the rest of the oil in a frying pan and gently fry the celery and red pepper until soft. Add the tomatoes, basil, seasoning and simmer for 10 minutes. Pour this mixture over the halibut. Cover the dish and place in the oven.

Bake for 15 minutes then remove cover and continue cooking for a further 7 minutes. Garnish with parsley before serving.

Note: Cod or haddock steaks can be substituted for the halibut in this recipe.

Fish with sorrel sauce

Serves 4 ★ W M E A

4 portions of fish (eg, cod, haddock, plaice)
30 g/1 oz Tomor margarine
chopped parsley to garnish

For the sauce:
30 g/1 oz Tomor margarine
120 g/4 oz sorrel leaves, finely chopped
1½ tbsp rice flour (use millet flour if following the arthritis exclusion diet)
300 ml/½ pint chicken stock (see page 90)
seasoning

Place the fish on the grill pan, dot with Tomor, and grill for about 6 minutes on each side – the fish should be cooked through, but not allowed to go dry. Keep warm.

Make the sauce by melting the margarine in a pan and adding the chopped sorrel. Cook the sorrel gently until it is soft. Add the flour, stirring well. Gradually add the stock, stirring all the time. Continue stirring until the sauce has thickened. Then add the seasoning.

Place the fish in a warmed serving dish and garnish with parsley. Serve with the sorrel sauce.

Cheese and fruit nut loaf (*top*, see page 67); Fruit and nut snack (*below left*, see page 67); Gram flour pancakes with savoury pancake filling (*below right*, see page 65)

Fish curry

Serves 2 ★ W M E

1 tbsp soya oil
4–5 tsp wheat-free curry powder
75 g/2½ oz red pepper, coarsely chopped
2 frozen cod steaks (120 g/4 oz each)
6–8 tomatoes, roughly chopped
150 g/5 oz fresh or frozen peas or runner beans
1–2 tbsp water (if necessary)
2 tsp creamed coconut (Sharwood's)
2 tsp garam masala

Heat the oil in a frying pan and fry the curry powder and the chopped red pepper. Move the pepper to one side of the pan and fry the cod steaks for 4–5 minutes on each side, or until they are thawed through. Add the chopped tomatoes and their juice, then the prepared peas or beans. Flake the fish into bite-size pieces and continue to simmer the mixture until all the ingredients are cooked, adding the extra water if necessary.

Towards the end of the cooking time, stir in the creamed coconut. Immediately before serving sprinkle on and stir in the garam masala.

West Country fish

Serves 2 ★ W M E A

2 mackerel, cleaned, washed and dried
200–250 g/7–9 oz cooking apples (unprepared weight)
seasoning
knob of Tomor margarine
150 ml/¼ pint apple juice

Preheat the oven to 180°C/350°F/gas 4.

Place fish in a shallow ovenproof dish. Peel the apples and flake them into the fish dish. Add seasoning and dot the fish with Tomor. Pour the apple juice round them.

Cover the dish with aluminium foil and bake in the oven for 30 minutes, basting once. Serve immediately.

Fish cakes

See photograph, page 69

W M E A

Makes 10–12 fish cakes

450 g/1 lb potatoes
450 g/1 lb white fish
30 g/1 oz Tomor margarine
2 tbsp milk substitute
2 tbsp finely chopped parsley
seasoning
millet flakes for coating
sunflower oil for frying

Boil the potatoes in lightly salted water until they are fairly soft and ready to mash. Gently cook the fish in sufficient salted water to cover, drain, remove the skin and bones and flake the flesh. Mash together the potatoes, fish, Tomor and milk substitute. Add the parsley and seasoning and mix well. Mould the mixture into round flat cakes and gently roll the cakes in the millet flakes until they are evenly coated.

Heat the oil in a frying pan. Fry the fish cakes for about 4 minutes on each side until golden brown.

MEAT

Tempting tornado

See photograph, page 82

★ W M E

Serves 2

280–340 g/10–12 oz braising steak
1 clove garlic, thinly sliced
6–8 tomatoes
3 medium carrots, sliced
½ medium green pepper, cored, seeded and chopped
420 g/15 oz cooked red kidney beans
seasoning
1 tsp chilli powder

Cut the steak into medium size cubes. Place the cubes in a heavy metal casserole and gently brown on top of the cooker. Enough fat and fluid will come out of the meat to stop it from burning if you keep the heat low. Add the garlic to the meat. Chop the tomatoes and add them, together with their juice. Then add the chopped carrots and green pepper. Using a slotted spoon, lift the beans from their juice and add them to the casserole. Stir in the seasoning and chilli powder and mix thoroughly.

Cover the casserole and simmer gently until the meat is cooked – a further 30–40 minutes – before serving.

Yorkshire potted beef

[★] [W] [M] [E]

225 g/8 oz beef steak (leg of beef is fine)
½ tsp ground mace
seasoning
30 g/1 oz Tomor margarine

Cut the beef into very small pieces. Place these in a pan with the smallest quantity of water necessary to enable you to simmer the beef for 1½ hours, or until it is really tender.

Remove the meat from the pan, retaining the stock that has formed during cooking. Allow the meat to cool and then run it through the mincer twice. Next add the mace, seasoning and sufficient of the jellied stock to achieve a firm yet moist consistency. Press into a mould, and seal with melted Tomor.

Arabian lamb

Serves 6

[★] [W] [M] [E]

1.8–2 kg/4–4½ lb leg of lamb (ask the butcher to bone it for you)

For the coating:
2 tbsp ground coriander
2 tbsp ground cumin
1 tbsp mild paprika
1 tbsp brown sugar
1 tsp freshly ground black pepper
1 large clove garlic
a little salt
4 tbsp olive oil

Four to five hours before you want to start roasting the meat, combine the coriander, cumin, paprika, brown sugar and pepper. Crush the garlic with a little salt and add this to the mixture with the olive oil. Mix thoroughly, then use to rub all over the inside and outside of the leg of lamb. Leave to allow the flavours to soak into the meat.

Preheat the oven to 220°C/425°F/gas 7.

Calculate the cooking time at 20 minutes per 450 g/1 lb and 20 minutes over. Cook the lamb, basting three or four times.

Serve with turmeric rice (see page 57) and a green salad. The cooking juices may be served with the lamb once you have skimmed off the fat.

Lamb paprika

Serves 4 ★ W M E

900 g/2 lb best end of neck of lamb chops
a little olive oil
2 sticks celery, finely chopped
225 g/8 oz tomatoes, skinned and chopped
1 tbsp chopped parsley
2 tbsp paprika pepper
200 ml/6½ fl oz water
seasoning
1 tsp basil
150 g/5 oz goat's yoghurt

Trim excess fat off the meat.

Heat a little olive oil in a pan. Lightly brown the chops in the oil. Remove the chops from the pan and add the celery. Sauté for a few minutes. Add the tomatoes, parsley, paprika, water and seasoning. Mix well. Return the chops to the pan and sprinkle the basil over the top. Gently bring to the boil, cover and simmer for 1½ hours.

Just before serving stir in the yoghurt, reheat but do not allow to boil. Check seasoning and serve.

Stuffed shoulder of lamb

Serves 4–6 ★ W M E

For the stuffing:
2 tbsp olive oil
120 g/4 oz lamb's liver, diced
1 stick celery, finely chopped
1 clove garlic, crushed
75 g/2½ oz cooked rice
60 g/2 oz raisins or sultanas
1 tbsp mixed dried herbs

1.35 kg/3 lb boned shoulder of lamb
2 sprigs rosemary
watercress to garnish

Preheat the oven to 180°C/350°F/gas 4.

Heat the oil in a pan and add the diced liver, celery and crushed garlic. Fry for a few minutes. Place the rice, raisins (or sultanas) and herbs in a large bowl. Add the fried ingredients and mix well. Leave to cool.

Stuff the lamb with the mixture, securing with skewers or stitching. Place the lamb in a roasting dish with the sprigs of rosemary on top. Roast in the oven for 1½–2 hours, until the lamb is cooked to your liking.

Drain off all the fat and place the stuffed lamb on a serving dish, garnished with watercress.

Thatched pork chops

See photograph, page 91

Serves 4 ★ W M E

4 pork chops
2 sticks celery, sliced
2 medium cooking apples, peeled, cored and sliced
30 g/1 oz granulated sugar
2.5 cm/1 in fresh ginger, peeled and grated
180 ml/6 fl oz water
30 g/1 oz brown sugar

Preheat the oven to 180°C/350°F/gas 4.

Lightly fry the chops in a heavy-bottomed frying pan. Place them in a shallow ovenproof dish. Fry the celery in the fat from the pork. Add the apples, sprinkle the white sugar and ginger on to the apples. Add the water, gently bring to the boil and simmer over a low heat for a few minutes. Arrange the apple mixture on top of the chops. Cover with foil and cook in the oven for 50 minutes.

Remove the lid, sprinkle with brown sugar and return to the oven uncovered for 10 minutes to brown. Serve immediately.

Pork and apple pie

Serves 2 W M E

340 g/12 oz stewing pork
1 tbsp oil
1 clove garlic, crushed
1 onion, chopped
1 medium cooking apple, peeled, cored and chopped
2 tsp sultanas
seasoning
100 ml/3½ fl oz apple juice
450 g/1 lb potatoes, peeled and thinly sliced
20 g/1½ oz Tomor margarine

Preheat the oven to 180°C/350°F/gas 4.

Trim any fat off the pork and cut the meat into cubes. Heat the oil in a pan. Fry the pork, turning frequently, until it is brown on all sides. Transfer the pork cubes to an ovenproof dish or casserole. In a bowl, mix together the garlic, onion, apple, sultanas and seasoning. Arrange the mixture on top of the meat. Pour the apple juice over the meat and vegetables. Arrange the potato slices over the top and dot with the Tomor. Cover with a lid or foil and place in the oven.

Cook the pie for 1–1½ hours, then remove the lid or foil and cook for a further 30 minutes to brown the potato topping before serving.

Pork and pepper casserole

Serves 4 ★ W M E

450 g/1 lb stewing pork
30 g/1 oz rice flour
seasoning
2 tbsp sunflower oil
1 stick celery, chopped
2 green peppers, seeded and sliced
225 g/8 oz tomatoes, skinned and chopped
150 ml/¼ pint tomato juice
½ tsp marjoram

Preheat the oven to 180°C/350°F/gas 4.

Trim the fat off the pork and cut the meat into cubes. Sieve together the flour and seasoning and coat the pork cubes with this mixture. Heat half the oil in a frying pan and fry the pork until it is browned, turning frequently. Transfer the meat to a casserole.

Pour the remaining oil into the frying pan and fry the prepared celery and peppers until they are soft. Transfer to the casserole. Add the tomatoes, tomato juice and marjoram, to the meat and vegetables in the casserole, mixing well.

Bake in the oven for 1½ hours, or until the meat is tender.

Marinated pork

Serves 6 ★ W M E

4 tbsp olive or sunflower oil
2 cloves garlic, crushed
1 tsp thyme
1 sprig rosemary (or 1 tsp dried rosemary)
1 tsp chopped parsley
seasoning
150 ml/¼ pint apple juice
6 pieces of pork or pork chops

Combine the first seven ingredients in a polythene bag, then add the pork portions. Shake well, then seal the bag. Leave in the refrigerator for 24 hours. Shake the bag two or three times during this period.

Remove the meat from the marinade and grill for 20 minutes, turning once, basting frequently with the marinade.

Pressed tongue

★ W M E

1 ox tongue
6 peppercorns
2 sticks celery, chopped
1 carrot, chopped
2 cloves
1 bay leaf
water
parsley to garnish

Place the tongue in the pressure cooker. Cover with water, gradually bring to the boil, *without the lid on*, then drain.

Lift out the trivet, replace the tongue, and add the other ingredients. Pour in enough water to come half way up the sides of the pressure cooker.

Cook at high pressure for 15 minutes per 450 g/1 lb, then allow the pressure to reduce at room temperature. Lift out the tongue and while it is still warm remove the skin and any fat. Curl into a small basin. Cover with a weighted saucer. Retain the cooking liquid for use as stock.

Allow tongue to cool, then turn out and garnish with parsley before serving.

Oriental stuffed lamb

Serves 4 ★ W M E

1.35 kg/3 lb shoulder of lamb, boned and unrolled
seasoning
1 tbsp sunflower oil

For the stuffing:
225 g/8 oz uncooked brown rice
120 g/4 oz dried apricots, soaked and chopped
3 tbsp raisins
50 g/1½ oz pine kernels, lightly toasted
2 cloves garlic, crushed
½ tsp cinnamon
1 tsp coriander
1 tsp ground ginger
seasoning

Preheat the oven to 190°C/375°F/gas 5.

Spread out the lamb and season it inside and out. Set aside. Cook the rice (see page 33). Drain it well, place in a large bowl and add the apricots, raisins, pine kernels, garlic, cinnamon, coriander, ginger and seasoning. Mix well. Take the lamb and stuff a little of the rice mixture into the hole where the bone was. Sew up the hole with a needle and thread. Brush the lamb with the oil and roast for 30 minutes per 450 g/1 lb (stuffed weight) and 20 minutes extra.

When the lamb is cooked, place on serving dish and keep warm. Pour the fat away from the pan juices, then add the rest of the rice mixture and reheat it, adding a little water if necessary. Arrange this around the lamb and serve with a salad or green vegetables.

Bobotie

Serves 6 W M

3 tbsp sunflower oil
340 g/12 oz onions, chopped
4 cloves garlic, crushed
675 g/1½ lb minced lamb or beef
1 tsp ground turmeric
1 tbsp wheat-free curry powder
2 tbsp white wine vinegar
150 ml/¼ pint beef stock (see page 90)

→

Oriental stuffed lamb (*above*); Bobotie (*below*)

OVERLEAF: Fruity chicken (*top left and right*, see page 85); Prune-striped turkey (*below left*, see page 88)

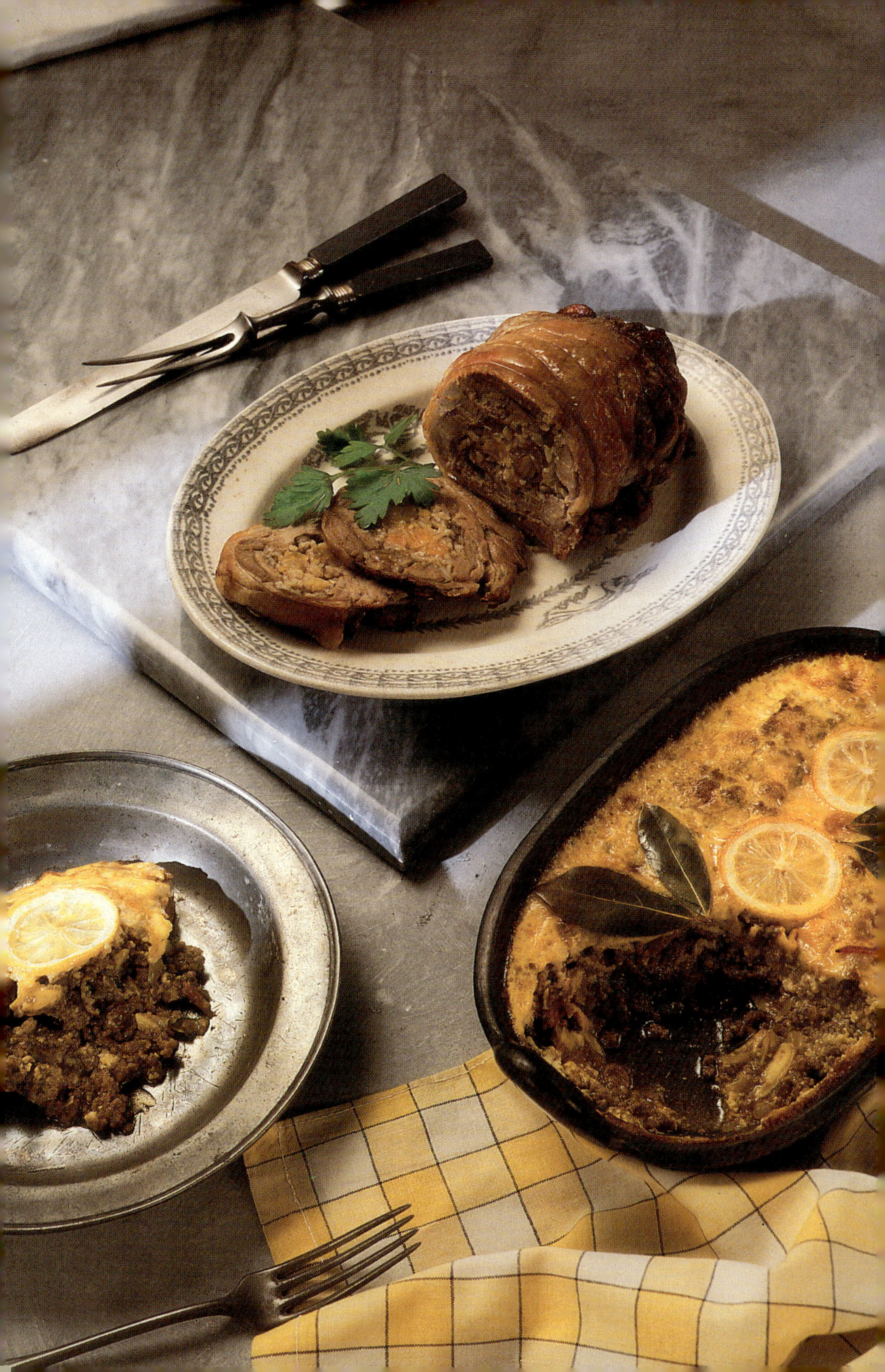

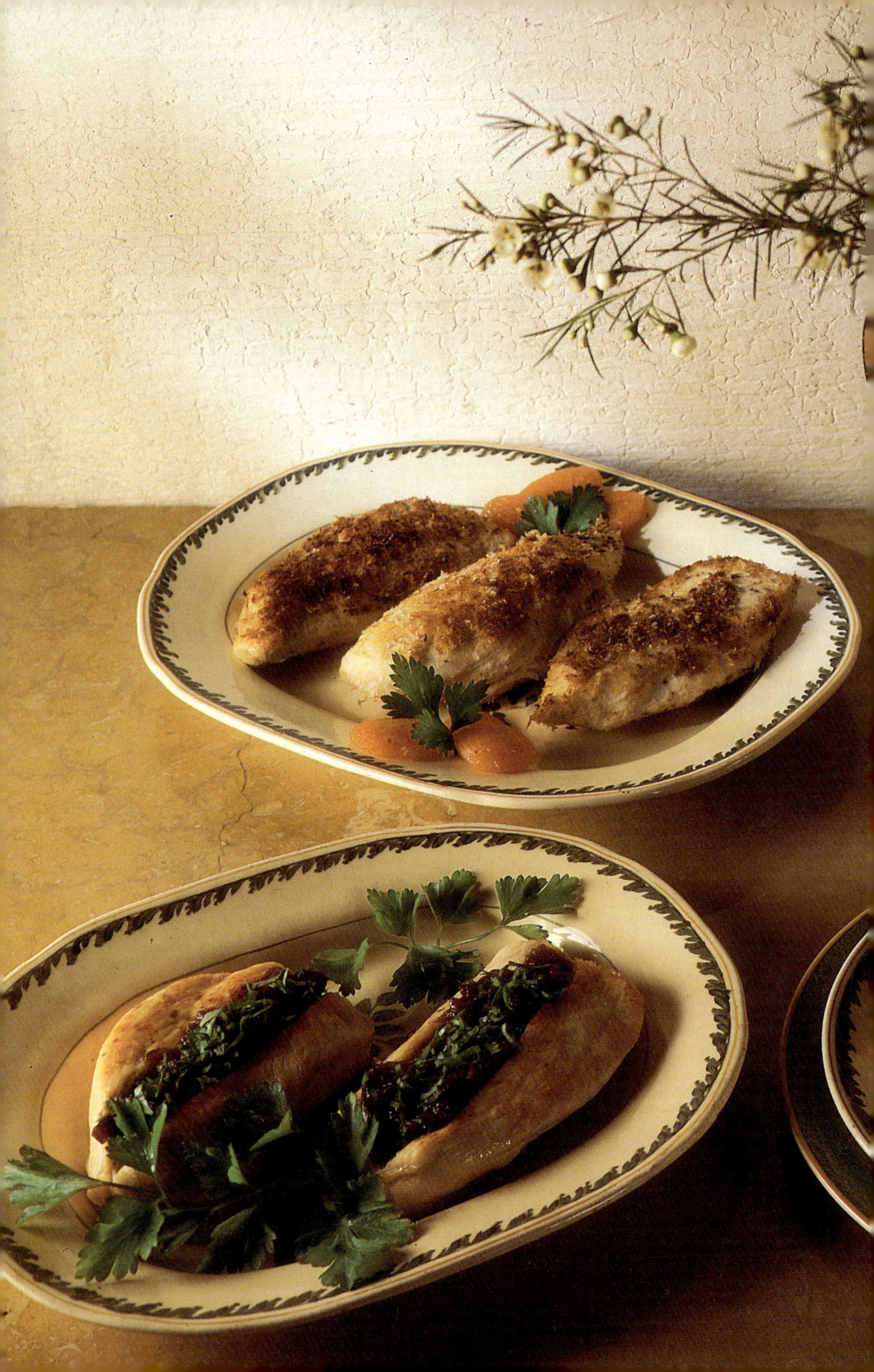

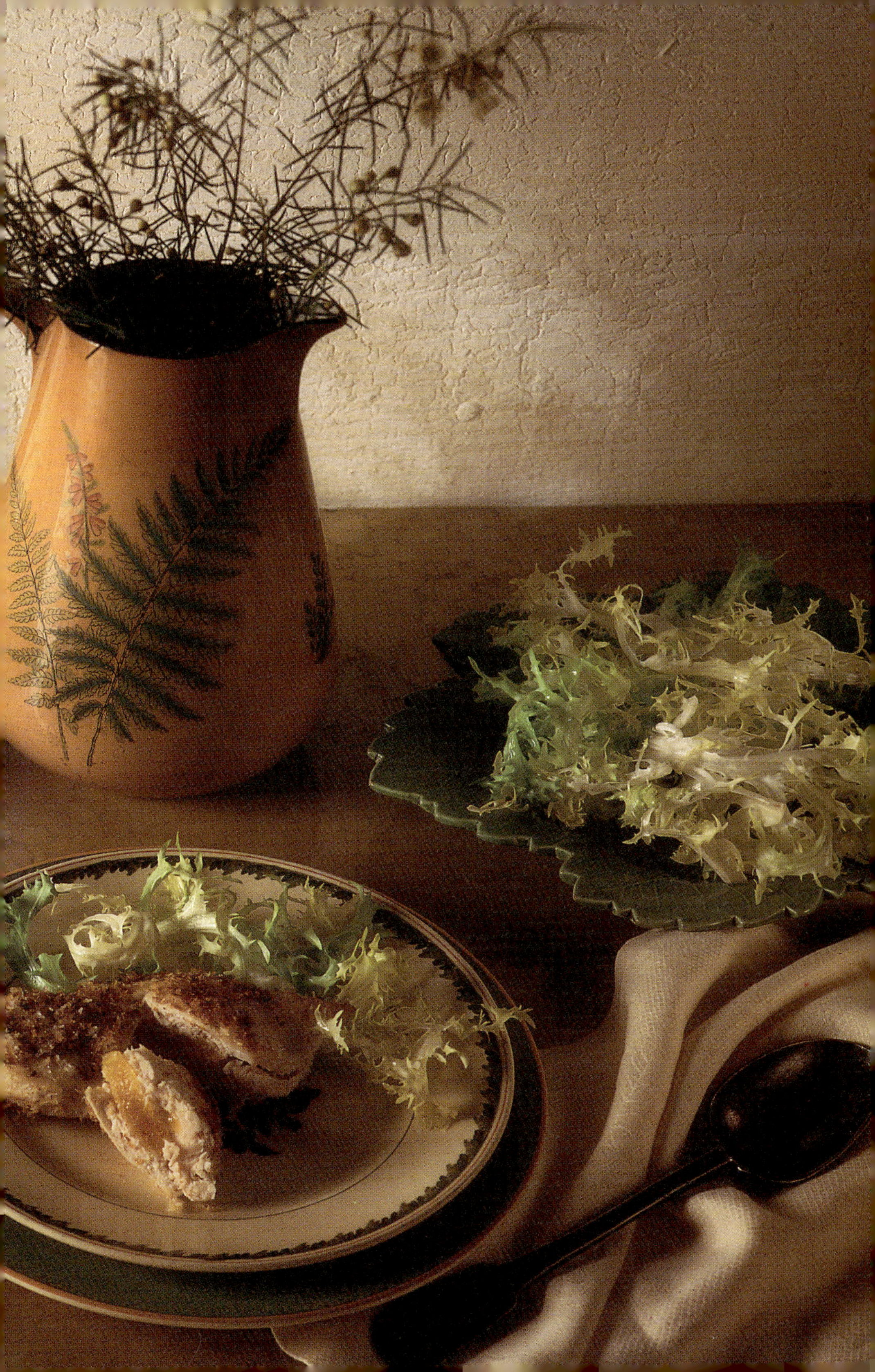

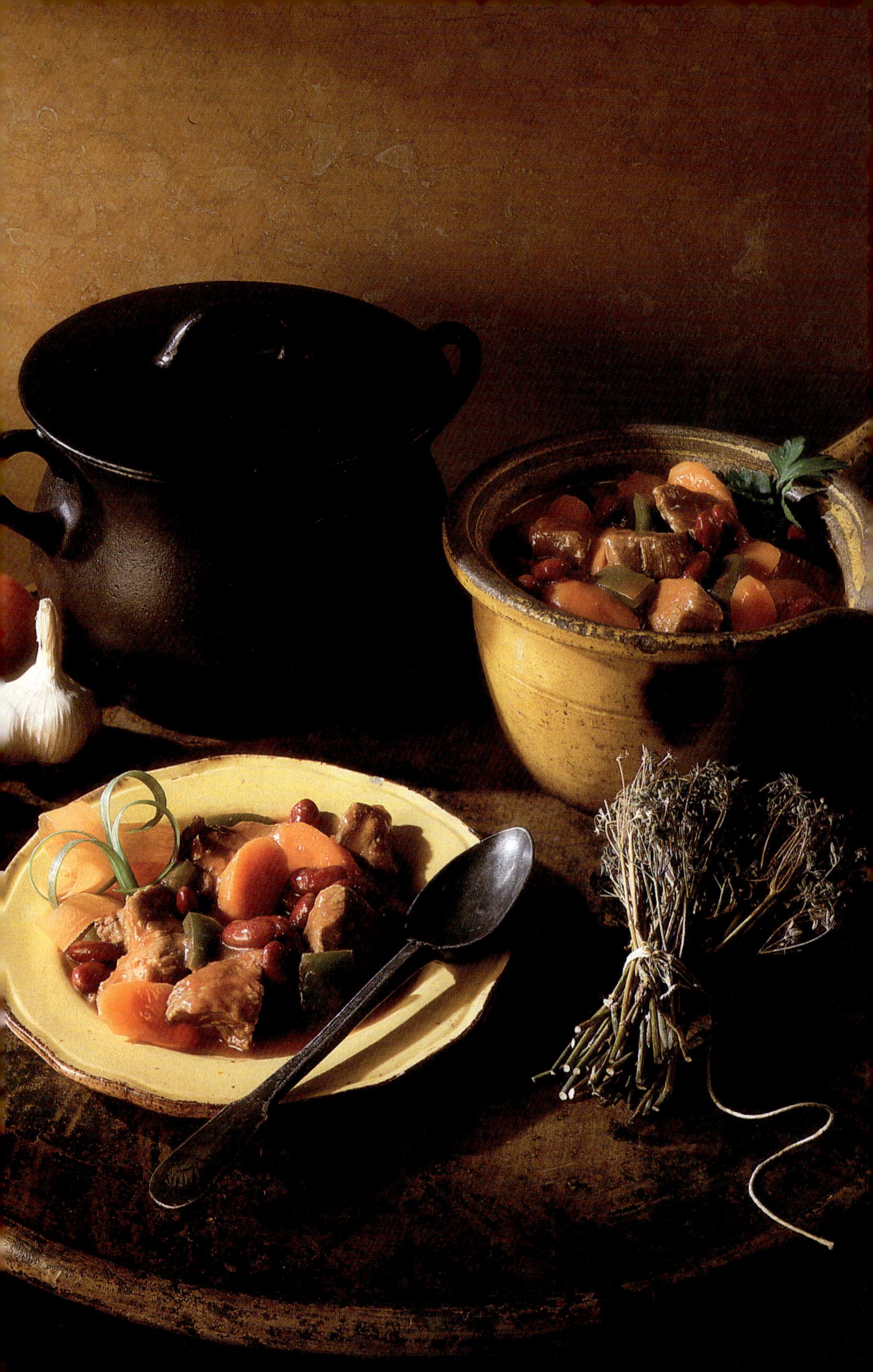

2 tomatoes, skinned and chopped
30 g/1 oz blanched almonds, chopped
60 g/2 oz sultanas
60 g/2 oz dried apricots, chopped
1 tbsp brown sugar
1 banana, chopped

For the custard topping:
2 eggs
300 ml/½ pint milk substitute
thin slices of lemon
3–4 fresh bay leaves

Preheat the oven to 180°C/350°F/gas 4.

Heat the oil in a large pan. Add the onions and garlic and cook until lightly browned. Add the minced lamb/beef and cook until the meat is browned. Drain off the oil. Add the turmeric, curry powder, vinegar, stock and tomatoes. Cook for 10 minutes uncovered. Add the almonds, sultanas, apricots, sugar and chopped banana. Mix well. Spoon the mixture into a shallow casserole dish.

To make the custard topping, beat the eggs with the milk substitute. Pour the custard over the top of the meat mixture. Arrange lemon slices and bay leaves in the custard. Bake in the oven for 30 minutes or until the custard is set.

Serve with rice and salad.

Note: If eggs cannot be tolerated, omit the custard topping.

Devilled kidneys

Serves 2 ★ W M E

1 tbsp wheat-free mustard powder
1 tsp wheat-free curry powder
1 tbsp rice flour
4 lamb's kidneys, skinned, cored and cut in half
60 g/2 oz Tomor margarine
2 tbsp tomato purée
150 ml/¼ pint water
seasoning

Sift the mustard powder, curry powder and rice flour together. Use this mixture to coat the kidneys. Melt the margarine in a pan and fry the kidneys for about 5 minutes, turning them frequently, until they are lightly browned. Stir in the tomato purée, water and seasoning. Bring to the boil. Cover the pan and simmer for 20 minutes or until the kidneys are tender.

Delicious served with brown rice and a mixed salad.

Tempting tornado (see page 73)

Corsican liver

Serves 4 [★] [W] [M] [E]

2 tbsp olive oil
1 clove garlic, crushed
1 green pepper, seeded and chopped
450 g/1 lb pig's or lamb's liver, sliced
450 g/1 lb tomatoes, skinned and seeded
1 tbsp brown rice miso
300 ml/½ pint hot water
1 tsp basil
½ tsp rosemary
½ tsp thyme
225 g/8 oz French beans, topped and tailed
chopped parsley to garnish

Preheat the oven to 200°C/400°F/gas 6.

Heat the oil in a frying pan. Gently fry the garlic and green pepper until soft. Remove from the pan with a slotted spoon and place in an ovenproof dish. Fry the liver slices for 2–3 minutes on each side. Remove with the slotted spoon and place on top of the garlic and pepper.

Put the tomatoes in the frying pan, dissolve the miso in the hot water and add to the pan with the herbs. Stir and simmer the mixture for 3–4 minutes.

Cut the French beans into 5 cm/2 in lengths and add these to the pan and bring to the boil. Pour the mixture over the liver. Cover the dish and bake in the oven for 30 minutes. Garnish with parsley and serve.

POULTRY

Stuffing for roast chicken

Makes enough stuffing for 1 large chicken [★] [W] [M] [E]

1 stick celery, finely chopped
2 cloves garlic, crushed
2 tbsp sunflower oil
60 g/2 oz uncooked long-grain white rice
150 ml/¼ pint hot water
120 g/4 oz mushrooms, sliced
30 g/1 oz sultanas
60 g/2 oz dried apricots, soaked and chopped
2 tsp tarragon
seasoning

Fry the celery and garlic in the oil for 2–3 minutes. Add the rice and sauté for a few more minutes. Pour in the hot water, stir, then simmer for 2–3 minutes until most of the water has been absorbed but the rice is still hard. Remove from the heat and mix in the remaining ingredients.

Allow to cool a little, then use to stuff the chicken.

Fruity chicken

See photograph, page 80

★ W M E A

Serves 4

170 g/6 oz dried apricots (or 4 bananas)
4 chicken breasts
85 g/3 oz desiccated coconut
85 g/3 oz Tomor margarine

Soak the apricots overnight and gently stew them for about 10 minutes. Alternatively, slice the bananas in half lengthways.

Stuff the chicken breasts with the apricots or 2 halves of banana each. Secure with wooden orange sticks or by stitching. Roll each chicken breast in the coconut.

Heat the Tomor in a frying pan. Fry the chicken breasts over a gentle heat for 2 minutes on each side. Remove from the pan and roll in coconut for a second time. Return to the pan and continue to fry gently for a further 8–10 minutes on each side.

Serve immediately.

Oriental chicken

★ W M E

Serves 4

50 g/1½ Tomor margarine
2 tbsp olive oil
450 g/1 lb chicken, cut into strips approximately 6 × 1½ cm (3 × ¾ in)
2.5 cm/1 in fresh ginger, peeled and grated
2 sticks celery, finely chopped
1 green pepper, seeded and cut into strips
8 carrots, cut into strips
120 g/4 oz button mushrooms, sliced
2 large tomatoes, skinned, seeded and sliced
280 g/10 oz beansprouts
½ tsp mixed herbs
seasoning
2 tbsp wheat-free tamari sauce

Heat the margarine and oil in a large, deep frying pan or wok. Fry the chicken and ginger, stirring all the time, for 3–4 minutes. Add the celery, pepper and carrots. Stir-fry for a further 4 minutes. Add the mushrooms and tomatoes. Continue cooking for 3 minutes, adding the beansprouts for the last minute. Add herbs and season. Add the tamari sauce and stir-fry for 1 minute more.

Serve at once, on its own or accompanied by brown rice.

Spicy chicken

Serves 4 ★ W M E

4 chicken pieces, skinned
2 tbsp chopped parsley
75 g/2½ oz Tomor margarine
120 g/4 oz runny honey
seasoning
1 tsp wheat-free curry powder
⅛ tsp each of: ground cumin, chilli powder, coriander, cinnamon, ginger, nutmeg and ground cloves
extra chopped parsley to garnish

Preheat the oven to 180°C/350°F/gas 4.

Place the chicken pieces in an overproof dish. Sprinkle the parsley over the chicken. Melt the Tomor in a pan and add the honey, seasoning and spices. Mix well. Pour over the chicken. Cover with foil and bake in the oven for 1 hour, removing the foil for the last 15 minutes.

Serve garnished with parsley. Brown rice goes very well with this dish.

Chicken in a coconut

Serves 4 ★ W M E A

1.8 kg/4 lb cooked chicken
4 fresh coconuts
2 red peppers, seeded and chopped
2 green peppers, seeded and chopped
120 g/4 oz button mushrooms, sliced
1 stick celery, finely chopped
seasoning

Preheat the oven to 160°C/325°F/gas 3.

Remove the skin and bones from the chicken and cut into bite-size pieces. Wash the coconuts. Saw off the tops and pour out the milk into a jug.

Place the peppers, mushrooms and celery in a pan and add the coconut milk. Season. Gradually bring the mixture to the boil and simmer gently until the peppers are soft, then stir in the chicken. Reheat, adding a little water if necessary.

Fill the coconuts with the chicken mixture. Seal the lids back on, using a paste of millet flour and water. Wrap in foil, place in the oven and cook for 1½ hours.

Note: Once cooked and left in the foil this dish will stay hot for 2–3 hours.

Chicken cormandel

Serves 4 ★ W M E

300 ml/½ pint soya milk
4 tbsp water
3 cloves garlic, crushed
120 g/4 oz desiccated coconut
1 tsp coriander
½ tsp cumin
450 g/1 lb leftover chicken or turkey
450 g/1 lb tomatoes, skinned, seeded and sliced
150 ml/¼ pint goat's yoghurt
seasoning
parsley and paprika to garnish

Place the milk in a pan. Add the water, garlic, coconut, coriander and cumin. Bring to the boil then simmer for 2–3 minutes. Set aside to cool.

Cut the chicken (or turkey) into bite-size pieces. Place in a serving dish with the prepared tomatoes.

When the coconut mixture is completely cold, drain through muslin or a fine sieve. Press down hard to extract all the milk. Mix the liquid with the yoghurt and season to taste. Pour over the chicken and tomatoes. Chill.

Just before serving, garnish with parsley and a little paprika.

Simple chicken and rice

Serves 2 ★ W M E

150 g/5 oz brown rice
450 ml/¾ pint water, very hot bu not boiling
20 g/½ oz brown rice miso
2 tsp tomato purée
seasoning
4 chicken drumsticks
1 bouquet garni
parsley to garnish

Place the rice in the bottom of a large thick-bottomed casserole with a tight-fitting lid. Add the hot water and stir in the miso, tomato purée and seasoning. Bring to the boil with the lid on. Stir well and add the chicken drumsticks and bouquet garni. Replace the lid and simmer until the rice has soaked up all the water (35–40 minutes), checking occasionally to make sure that it has not dried out.

Serve in the cooking dish, garnished with parsley. Spinach makes a good accompaniment to this dish.

Crispy chicken with herb tomatoes

Serves 2 ★ W M E

2 chicken joints
knob Tomor margarine at room temperature
seasoning
2 tomatoes
1 tsp granulated sugar
4 pinches mixed herbs
watercress to garnish

→

Place the chicken joints in the grill pan with the inner joint surface uppermost and grill until they are cooked on that side. Lift the grill pan out and turn the joints skin side uppermost. Spread the Tomor evenly over the joints, then rub in the seasoning. Halve the tomatoes and sprinkle the sugar and herbs on to the cut surfaces, together with a little seasoning. Place them on the grill pan around the chicken joints and grill until the second side of the chicken is cooked and the tomatoes are soft.

Serve garnished with watercress.

Chicken in mango sauce

Serves 4 ★ W M E A

4 chicken quarters
1 mango
1 pinch salt
2 tbsp water
1 tbsp mango chutney (Sharwood's)

Grill the chicken joints.

Meanwhile, halve the mango and scoop out the flesh, discarding the skin. Place the mango flesh in a pan with the salt and water. Gently stew until the mango is soft enough to mash – the consistency should be a bit firmer than apple sauce. Stir in the mango chutney.

Put the grilled chicken in a serving dish, pour the mango sauce over the top and serve immediately.

Prune-striped turkey

See photograph, page 80

Serves 2 ★ W M E A

4–5 prunes
2 turkey breast steaks
seasoning
knob of Tomor margarine (optional)
chopped parsley to garnish

Place the prunes in a pan and simmer, in the smallest quantity of water possible, until they go soft (about 5 minutes). Next, remove the prune stones and mash the flesh.

Place the turkey breasts on the grill pan, season and dot with Tomor (if required). Grill one side for 10 minutes. Before cooking the second side, make a cut into, but not all the way through, the uncooked side of the steak lengthways. Pack the prune purée into this slit, return to the grill and cook the second side for 5–10 minutes. Garnish with parsley and serve.

Duck with olives

Serves 4

☒ W M E

1.8 kg/4 lb duck
salt
2 cloves garlic, crushed
225 g/8 oz red pepper, seeded and chopped
120 g/4 oz button mushrooms, wiped but not peeled
4 medium tomatoes, skinned and seeded
seasoning
60 g/2 oz stuffed green olives

Preheat the oven to 180°C/350°F/gas 4.

Prick the skin of the duck all over and rub with salt. Roast the duck on a rack in the oven for 2 hours. Remove from tin and take off most of the fat. Keep the duck warm.

Place the roasting tin on the cooker and gently fry the garlic and pepper in a little of the cooking fat. Add the mushrooms and tomatoes. Cook over a low heat for 7 minutes. Season to taste.

Prepare the duck by dividing it into four portions. Place them in an ovenproof dish and cover with the pepper mixture. Cover and bake in the oven for 45 minutes. Add the olives 10 minutes before the end of the cooking time.

Marinated duck

Serves 2

☒ W M E

2 portions of duck
2.5 cm/1 in fresh ginger, peeled and grated
2 tbsp olive oil
2 tbsp runny honey
2 tbsp apple juice
1 tbsp wheat-free tamari sauce
watercress to garnish

Slash the skin of the duck in three or four places.

Make the marinade by mixing together the ginger, olive oil, honey, apple juice and tamari sauce. Pour the marinade over the duck and leave to marinate for at least 4 hours, turning frequently.

Grill the duck under a high heat for 25 minutes, turning once and basting four or five times with the marinade.

Alternatively, bake on a rack in the oven, again basting several times, for 40 minutes (oven temperature 200°C/400°F/gas 6).

Garnish with watercress and serve.

STOCKS, SAUCES AND JAMS

Stocks

★ W M E

Vegetable stock An economical substitute for stock is the water in which any allowed vegetables have been cooked.

Use vegetable leftovers and discards such as the outer leaves of cabbage or spinach. Wash and store in the refrigerator in a plastic bag. When ready to make stock, chop the vegetables, just cover with lightly salted water and boil slowly for 15 minutes to extract flavours, vitamins and minerals. Strain off the liquid and cool.

Meat or chicken stock Use the raw bones of any suitable meat or poultry. Cover the bones with lightly salted cold water, bring to the boil and simmer for 3 hours, or cook in a pressure cooker for 30 minutes. Strain off the liquid and allow to cool, then lift off fat.

Store any unused stock in the refrigerator, or freeze it.

Gravies

★ W M E

Vegetable purées can be used in place of conventional gravy mixes such as Bisto, stock cubes or instant gravies. For convenience the purées can be made in bulk and frozen in smaller quantities for later use.

Examples

1. Red cabbage and mushrooms with sea salt and black pepper cooked with a knob of Tomor margarine and a little water until soft, then put through a blender, makes a rich replacement for gravy.
2. Skinned tomatoes, leeks, basil and sugar cooked together until soft, then put through a blender, makes a sweet sauce, ideal for lamb and minced beef dishes.
3. Carrots, celery and leeks with parsley cooked until soft, then put through a blender, makes a good accompaniment to chicken, turkey or egg dishes.

Thatched pork chops (see page 76)

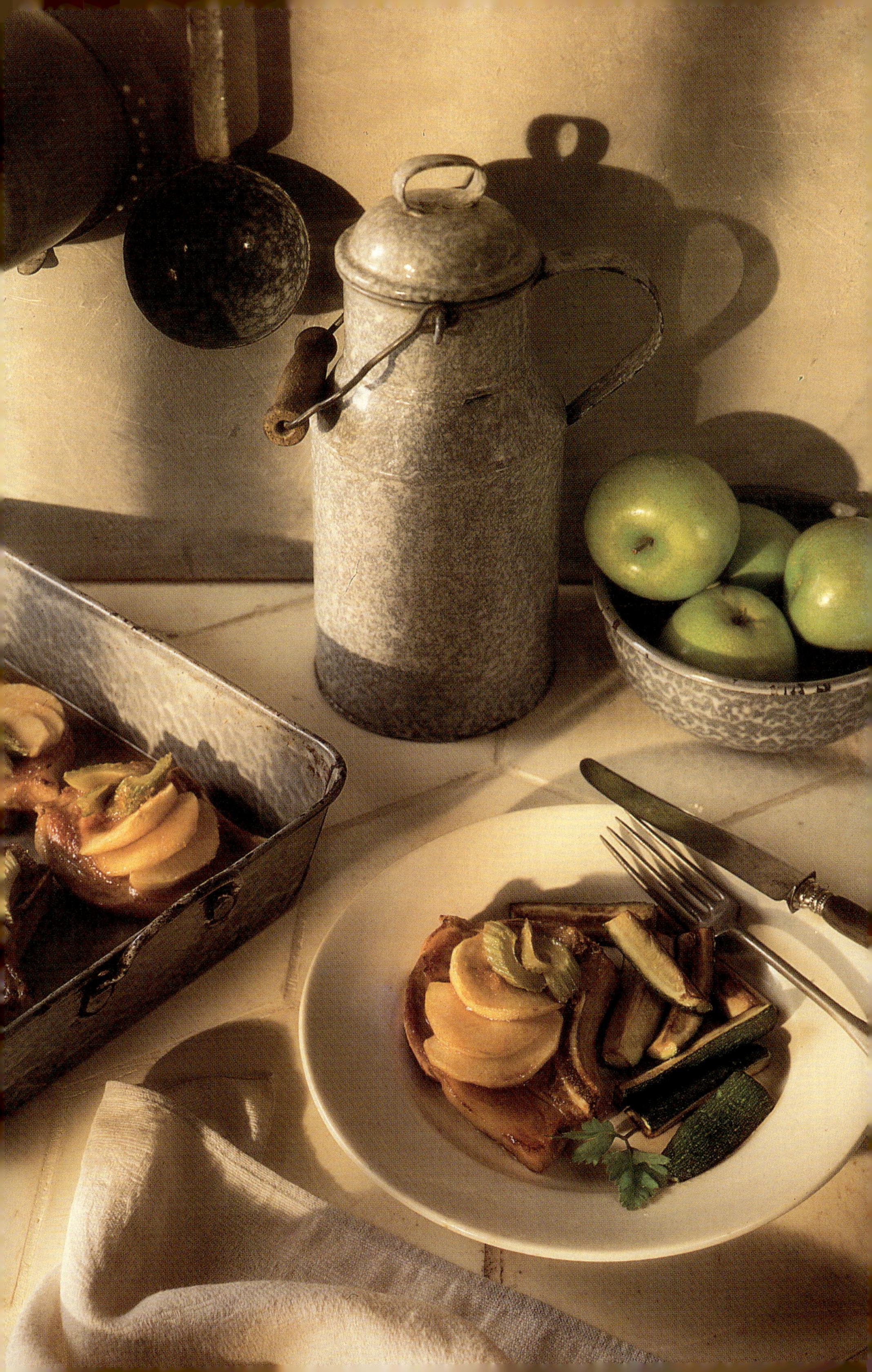

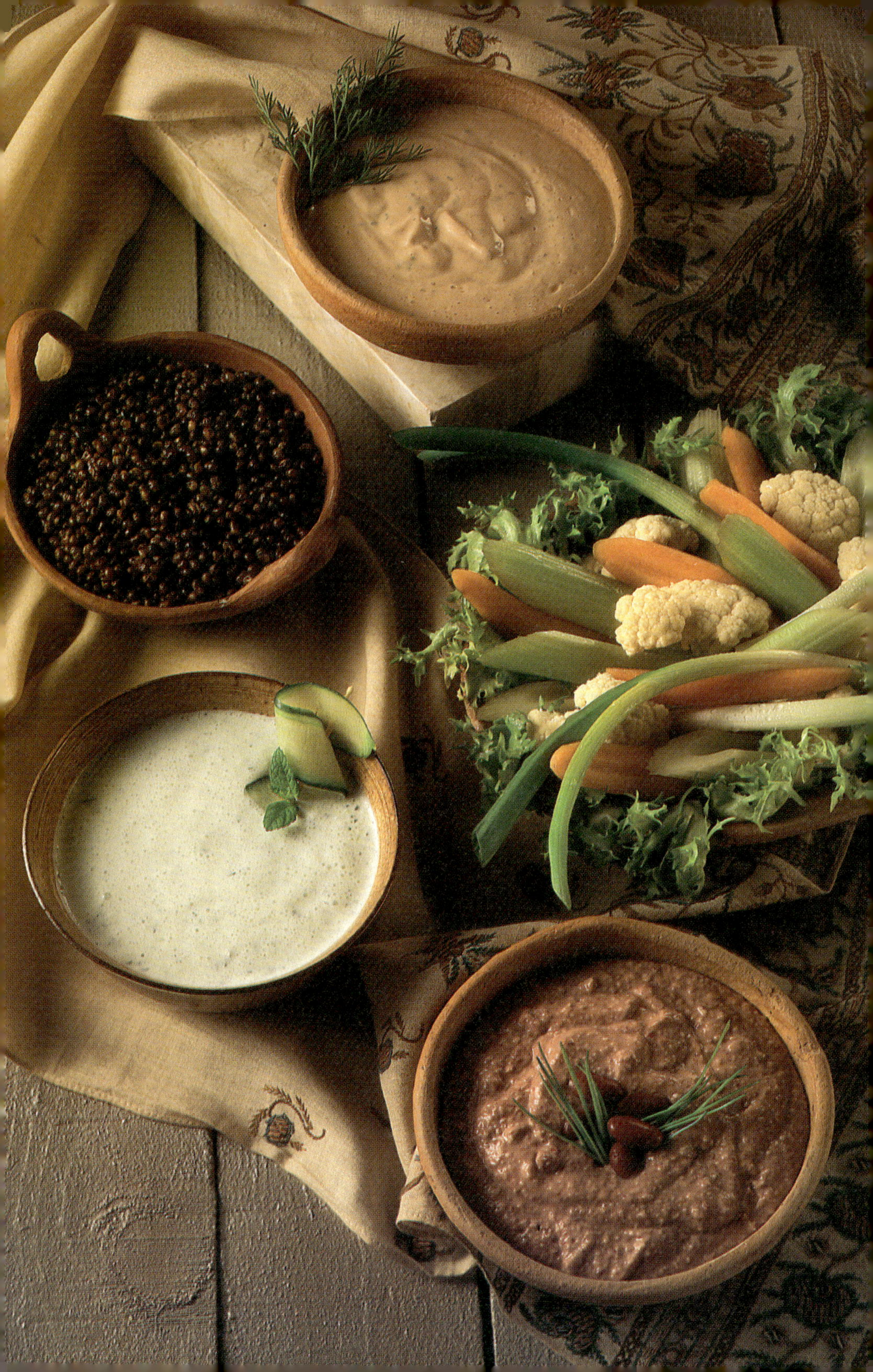

Green pepper sauce ★ W M E A

Makes approximately 300 ml/½ pint

340 g/12 oz green peppers, seeded and chopped
4 cloves garlic
7 tbsp safflower oil
1 tbsp apple juice
seasoning

Place the peppers in a pan with the garlic. Cover with water, bring to the boil and simmer for 10 minutes. Pour off the water and put the garlic and peppers in the liquidizer. Blend, pouring in the oil as you do so. Add the apple juice, and seasoning. Blend again.

Return the sauce to the pan and warm through very gently. Serve poured over poached fish or chicken.

Note: This sauce can be made into a delicious salad dressing by adding 6 cm/2½ in cucumber, chopped, and 2 tbsp goat's yoghurt when liquidizing.

Walnut raita

Serves 4 W M E

600 ml/1 pint goat's or ewe's yoghurt
60 g/2 oz shelled walnuts, broken roughly into pieces
2 tbsp finely chopped coriander
1 small onion, finely chopped
seasoning

Beat the yoghurt until smooth and creamy. Add all the other ingredients and mix well.

Good served with curries or other spicy dishes.

Coconut sauce

Serves 2 ★ W M E A

100 g/3½ oz creamed coconut (Sharwood's)
150 ml/¼ pint hot water

Crumble the creamed coconut into the hot water, and beat the mixture until it is smooth.

Serve chilled with baked apples (see page 116).

Blackcurrant jam

Makes 2.7 kg/6 lb jam ★ W M E

675 g/1½ lb blackcurrants, topped and tailed
1.1 l/2 pints water
1.58 kg/3½ lb preserving sugar

→

From the top: Tofu spread (see page 63); Deep fried mung beans (see page 64); Cucumber dip (see page 63); Bean and apple dip (see page 64)

Place the currants in a large pan with the water. Boil for 30 minutes. Add the sugar and boil rapidly for 10 minutes. Turn into warm jars and seal. Stored in a cool place, the jam keeps for over 1 year.

Note: It is very important to boil the mixture *very* rapidly after the sugar has been added or the jam will not set.

Raspberry or loganberry jam

Makes 1.4 kg/3 lb jam ★ W M E

900 g/2 lb raspberries or loganberries
½ tbsp water
760 g/1¾ lb preserving sugar

Place the raspberries (or loganberries) in a large pan with the water. Cook over a gentle heat until the berries are soft. Add the sugar and bring to the boil quickly. Boil very rapidly for 8 minutes.

Turn into warm dry jars and cover. Keeps for about 8 weeks.

Note: This jam is very good, but it must be boiled *very* fiercely after the sugar has been added.

Blackberry and apple jelly

Makes approximately 1.8 kg/4 lb jelly ★ W M E

1.35 kg/3 lb blackberries, stalks removed
675 g/1½ lb cooking apples
340 g/12 oz preserving sugar to every 600 ml/1 pint juice

Remove any stalks from the blackberries and rinse them. Place them in a large pan and cover with cold water. Bring to the boil and simmer until the berries are soft and the water is dark red. Drain through muslin or a fine sieve. The berries should be left draining overnight.

Cut the apples into quarters. Place in a pan and just cover with cold water. Bring to the boil and simmer until the apples are very tender. Drain in the same way as the blackberries, again leaving them overnight to obtain as much juice as possible.

Mix and measure the juices. Place in a large pan with 340 g/12 oz sugar to each 600 ml/1 pint of juice. Boil quickly until setting point is reached (105°C/221°F, test with a sugar thermometer). This should take approximately 30 minutes.

Turn into warm dry jars and seal.

Plum jam

Makes about 4.5 kg/10 lb jam ★ W M E

2.7 kg/6 lb plums
900 ml/1½ pints water
2.7 kg/6 lb preserving sugar

Wash the plums and remove the stones. Put the plums in a large pan, add the water and simmer gently until the plums are soft. Then add the sugar to the pan and boil the mixture rapidly until the setting point is reached (105°C/221°F-when tested with a sugar thermometer).

Pot and cover.

BREAD AND PASTRY

Baking powder

Baking powder contains starch such as rice flour, cornflour and frequently wheat flour. Always check the list of ingredients on any bought baking powder to make sure it is safe for you. Commercial wheat-free brands currently available in the UK are the Co-op's and Sainsbury's, and from health food shops, Bestoval, Food Watch, Hinton and Rite-Diet. If you are unable to find a suitable baking powder you can make your own:

Homemade wheat-free baking powder

60 g/2 oz rice flour
60 g/2 oz bicarbonate of soda
130 g/4½ oz cream of tartar

Sift the ingredients together at least three times. Store in an air-tight container in a dry place.

Note: The recipes in this book are made with commercial wheat-free baking powder. If using homemade, slightly more is required, eg, if 2 tsp baking powder is stated in the recipe, use 3 tsp home-made powder.

Date and walnut loaf

See photograph, page 102

For a 900 g/2 lb loaf tin W M

225 g/8 oz chopped dates
1 tsp bicarbonate of soda
1 pinch salt
300 ml/½ pint hot water
280 g/10 oz rice flour
1 tsp wheat-free baking powder (see page 95)
120 g/4 oz Tomor margarine
60 g/2 oz shelled walnuts, chopped
120 g/4 oz soft brown sugar
1 egg

Preheat oven to 180°C/350°F/gas 4.

Place dates, bicarbonate of soda and salt in a bowl and pour the hot water over the top. Leave to cool.

Sift the flour with the baking powder twice. Rub the margarine into the flour. Drain the dates and mix them into the flour along with the walnuts and sugar. Beat the egg and add to the flour mixture.

Grease a 900 g/2 lb loaf tin with Tomor, fill with the mixture and bake for 1½ hours. Turn out on to a wire tray to cool.

Note: Currants or raisins can be substituted for dates. This loaf cuts much better if left for a day.

Simple banana loaf

For a 900 g/2 lb loaf tin W M

200 g/7 oz millet flour
2 tsp wheat-free baking powder (see page 95)
½ tsp bicarbonate of soda
75 g/2½ oz Tomor margarine
135 g/4½ oz caster sugar
4 ripe bananas, mashed
2 eggs

Preheat the oven to 190°C/375°F/gas 5.

Sift the millet flour, baking powder and bicarbonate of soda together. Rub in the margarine until well mixed. Add the sugar and bananas. Mix well. Beat the eggs and add them to the other ingredients. Mix again.

Grease a 900 g/2 lb loaf tin with Tomor. Turn the mixture into it and bake for 1 hour.

Turn out on to a wire rack to cool.

Note: Sultanas or chopped crystallized ginger can be added to this recipe for variation.

Banana bread

For a 900 g/2 lb loaf tin [W] [M]

225 g/8 oz rice flour
2 tsp wheat-free baking powder (see page 95)
½ tsp salt
120 g/4 oz Tomor margarine
170 g/6 oz caster sugar
60 g/2 oz shelled walnuts, roughly chopped
450 g/1 lb ripe bananas
2 eggs

Preheat the oven to 180°C/350°F/gas 4.

Sift the flour, baking powder and salt into a bowl. Cut the margarine into pieces and rub it into the flour mixture. Add the sugar and nuts. In a separate bowl, mash the bananas, then beat the eggs into the mashed bananas. Add the flour/margarine mixture and mix very thoroughly.

Grease a 900 g/2 lb loaf tin, fill with the mixture and bake for 1½ hours. Remove from oven and cool on a wire tray. This mixture makes a moist loaf.

Variation You can add candied peel and the grated rind of half an orange (if allowed) to this recipe.

Coconut loaf

For a 450 g/1 lb loaf tin [W] [M]

120 g/4 oz Tomor margarine
120 g/4 oz caster sugar
2 eggs
170 g/6 oz rice flour
1½ tsp wheat-free baking powder (see page 95)
3 tbsp desiccated coconut
2 tbsp soya milk
a little icing sugar

Preheat the oven to 180°C/350°F/gas 4.

Place the margarine and sugar in a mixing bowl and cream them together. Beat in one of the eggs.

Sift the rice flour with the baking powder twice, then fold half the flour into the Tomor/sugar/egg mixture. Mix in the other egg and then fold in the remaining flour. Add the coconut and the soya milk. Mix well.

Grease a 450 g/1 lb loaf tin with Tomor and fill it with the mixture. Bake for 1¼ hours.

Turn out on to a wire tray to cool. Dust with icing sugar.

Apple and walnut loaf

For a 900 g/2 lb loaf tin W M

120 g/4 oz Tomor margarine
120 g/4 oz caster sugar
2 eggs
225 g/8 oz millet flour
1 tbsp wheat-free baking powder (see page 95)
1 pinch salt
1 tsp mixed spice
1 cooking apple, peeled, cored and chopped
85 g/3 oz walnuts

Preheat the oven to 180°C/350°F/gas 4.

Place the margarine and sugar in a large mixing bowl and cream them together. Beat the eggs and add them to the mixture. Mix well.

Sift the flour, baking powder, salt and spice together twice and stir into the mixture in the bowl. Add the apple and walnuts. Mix again.

Grease a 900 g/2 lb loaf tin with Tomor. Turn the mixture into the tin and bake for 1½ hours.

Turn out on to a wire rack to cool.

Yoghurt and sultana scones

See photograph, page 102

Makes 16 scones ★ W M E

250 g/9 oz millet flour
4 tsp wheat-free baking powder (see page 95)
50 g/1½ oz Tomor margarine
60 g/2 oz caster sugar
60 g/2 oz sultanas
150 ml/¼ pint goat's yoghurt
a little soya milk
30 g/1 oz demerara sugar

Preheat the oven to 220°C/425°F/gas 7.

Sift the flour and baking powder together into a mixing bowl. Rub in the margarine. Add the sugar and sultanas. Add the yoghurt and mix until the mixture can be moulded into a ball.

Dust a board and rolling pin with a little millet flour and roll out the mixture to a thickness of about 1.5 cm/¾ in. Cut into rounds with a 3 cm/1¼ in cutter. Brush the rounds with soya milk and place them on a baking tray that has been greased with Tomor. Sprinkle the scones with demerara sugar and bake for 7 minutes.

Pâte sucrée

Sufficient to line a 19 cm/7½ in flan tin W M

50 g/1½ oz ground almonds
50 g/1½ oz rice flour
50 g/1½ oz caster sugar
pinch salt
2 egg yolks
50 g/1½ oz Tomor margarine
a little water (if necessary)

Preheat the oven to 190°C/375°F/gas 5.

Sift the dry ingredients together to make a pyramid in the base of a mixing bowl. Make a hollow in the middle of the pyramid and tip the egg yolks into it, together with the Tomor, chopped into pieces. Working rapidly with your fingertips, rub the ingredients together, making a firm dough. Add a little water if necessary to bind the ingredients. When well blended, leave the dough in the refrigerator for 10 minutes.

Dust a board and rolling pin with rice flour. Grease a 19 cm/7½ in flan tin with Tomor. Remove the dough from the refrigerator and roll it out. Use it to line the flan tin and bake blind for 10–15 minutes.

The pâte sucrée can then be used immediately, filled with your chosen filling, or it will keep for a couple of days in the refrigerator. Alternatively, it can be frozen and kept for later use.

CAKES AND BISCUITS

Eggless fruit cake

For a 20 cm/8 in diameter cake tin ★ W M E

450 ml/¾ pint water
120 g/4 oz currants
120 g/4 oz raisins
225 g/8 oz Tomor margarine
170 g/6 oz demerara sugar
120 g/4 oz millet flour
120 g/4 oz rice flour
1 tbsp wheat-free baking powder (see page 95)
1 tsp bicarbonate of soda
1 tsp mixed spice

Preheat the oven to 190°C/375°F/gas 5.

Place the water, currants, raisins, margarine and sugar in a pan and bring to the boil. Simmer for 5 minutes. Leave to cool.

Sift the millet flour, rice flour, baking powder, bicarbonate of soda and mixed spice together three times.

When the ingredients in the pan are quite cold mix them with the flour mixture until thoroughly combined.

Grease a loose-bottomed 20 cm/8 in cake tin with Tomor. Fill with the mixture and bake for 2 hours.

Leave the cake to cool in the tin for a few minutes before turning it on to a wire tray.

Coconut and raspberry Swiss roll

For a 23 × 15 cm(9 × 6 in) Swiss roll tin W M

2 large eggs
100 g/3½ oz caster sugar
60 g/2 oz millet flour
4 tbsp desiccated coconut
6 tbsp raspberry jam (see page 94)

Preheat the oven to 200°C/400°F/gas 6.

Whisk the eggs and 75 g/2½ oz of the sugar over a pan of hot water until thick and creamy. Remove from the heat and whisk until cold.

→

Coconut and raspberry Swiss roll (*left*); Honey cake (*right*, see page 105); Ginger biscuits (*centre*, see page 109)

OVERLEAF LEFT: Date and walnut loaf (*above*, see page 96); Yoghurt and sultana scones (*below*, see page 98)

OVERLEAF RIGHT: Blackcurrant and tofu whip (*top*, see page 116); Millet and hazelnut ice (*centre*, see page 117); Carob ice cream (*below*, see page 117)

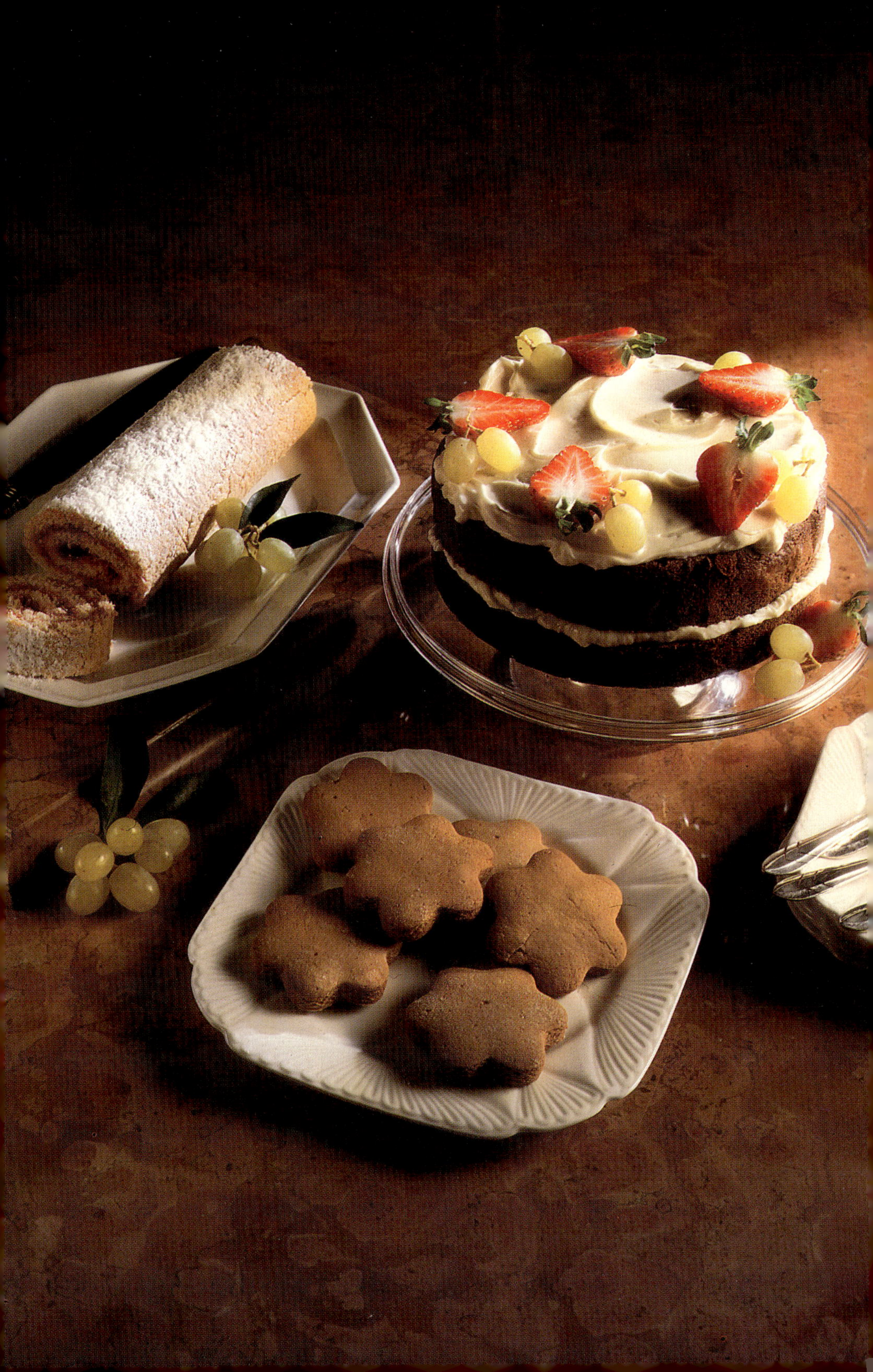

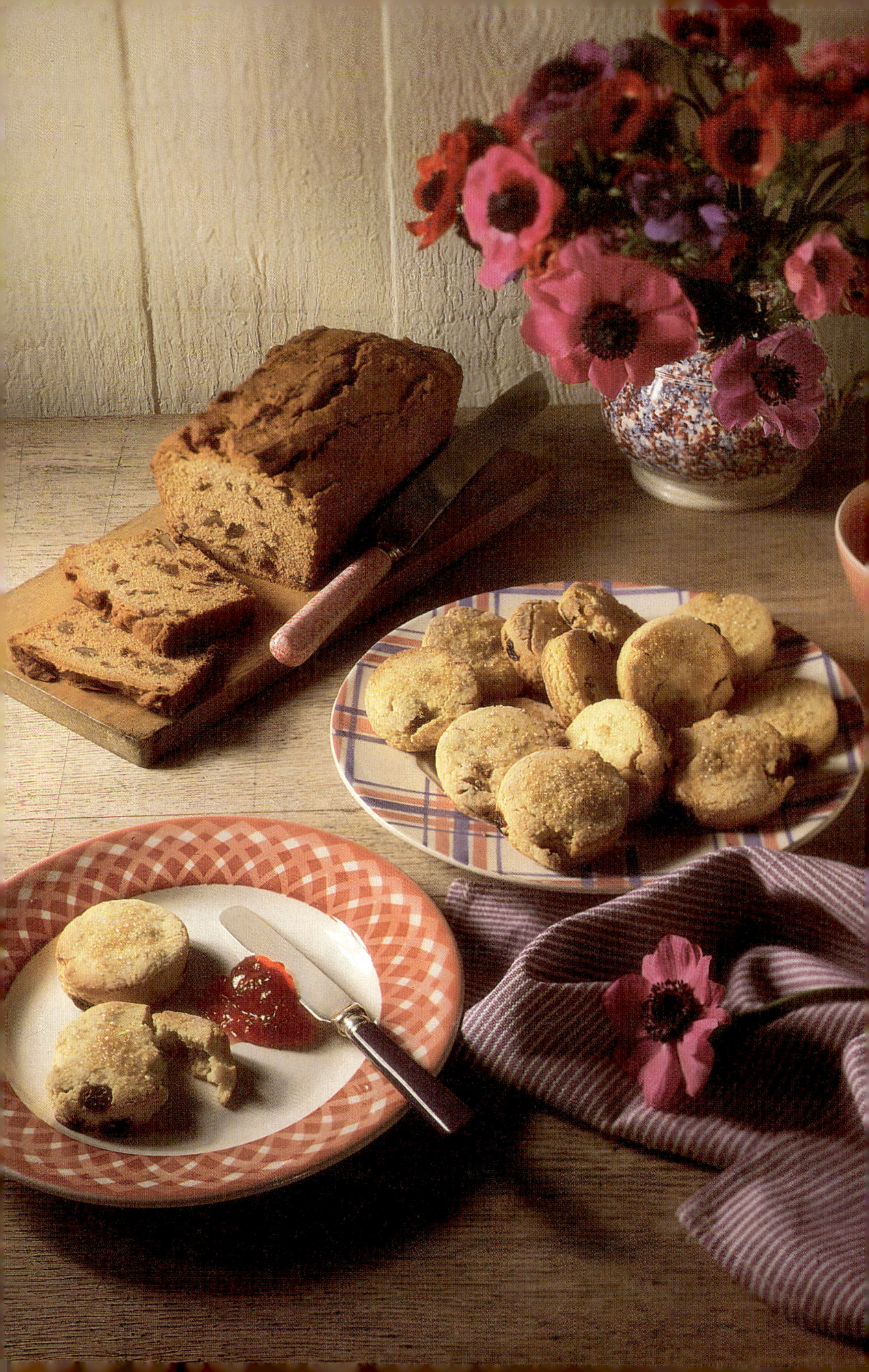

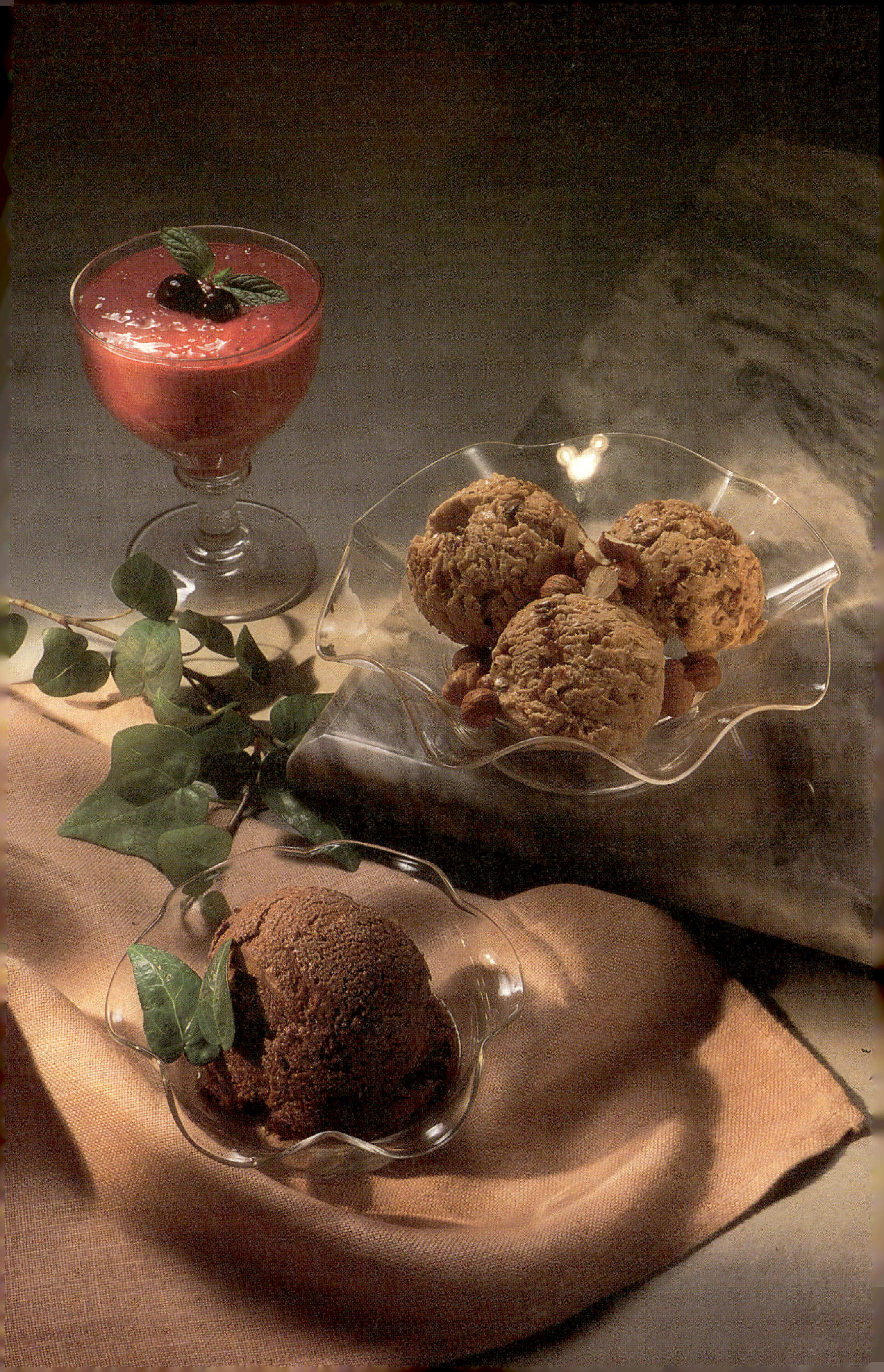

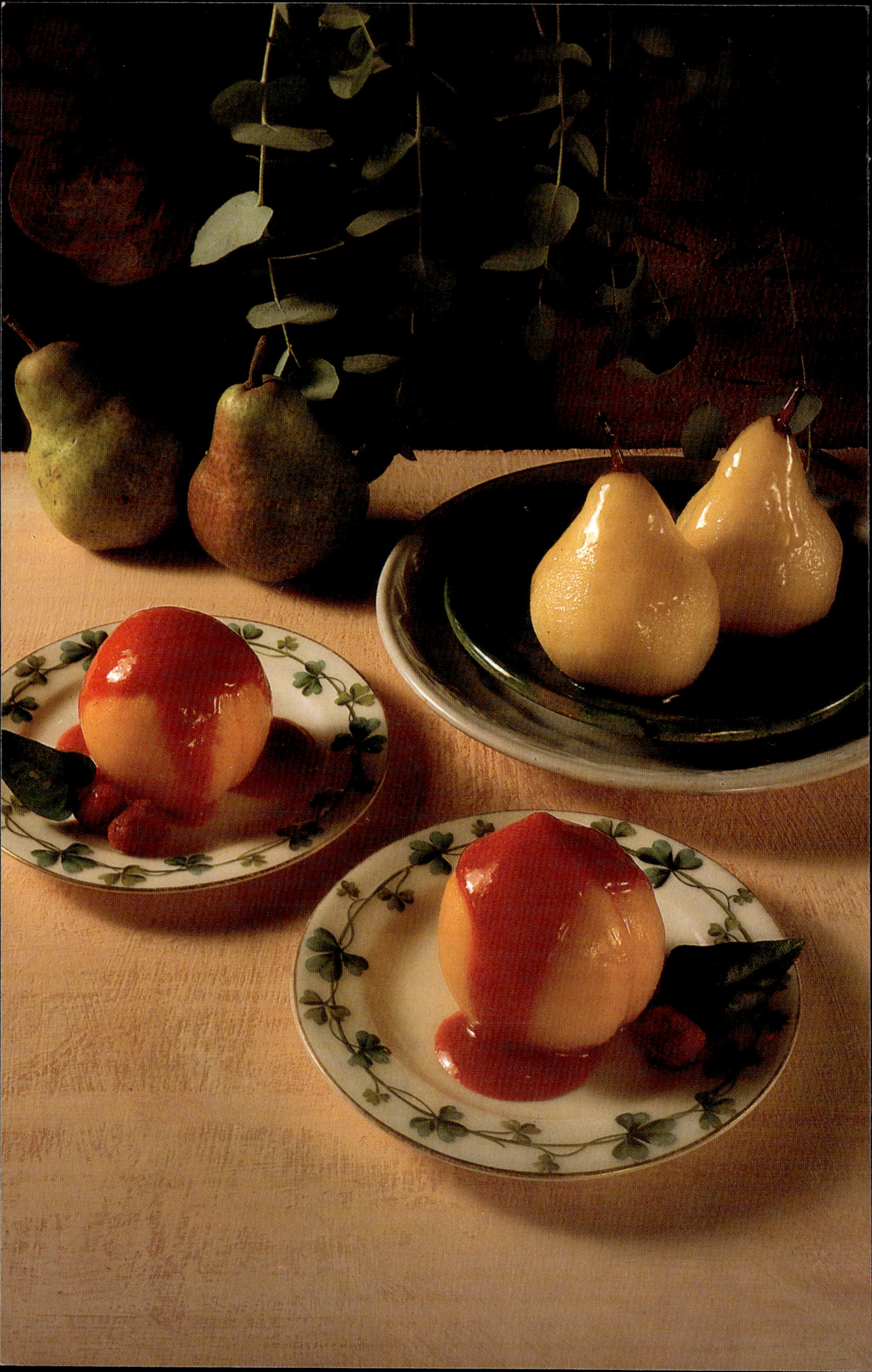

Sift the flour through a fine sieve three times. Fold the sifted flour into the egg mixture using a metal spoon. Then fold in 3 tbsp of the coconut in the same way.

Line and grease a 23 × 15 cm (9 × 6 in) Swiss roll tin, using Tomor. Turn the mixture into the tin and bake for 8–10 minutes, or until the top is light brown and springs back when gently pushed with a finger.

Turn the sponge on to greaseproof paper and spread with the warmed jam. Roll up, using the greaseproof paper to help you. Dust with the remaining icing sugar and coconut.

Best eaten on the same day.

Rice sponge

For a 15 cm/6 in diameter cake tin W M

120 g/4 oz Tomor margarine
120 g/4 oz granulated sugar
2 eggs
vanilla essence to taste
170 g/6 oz ground rice
1½ tsp wheat-free baking powder (see page 95)
1 pinch salt

Preheat the oven to 180°C/350°F/gas 4.

Grease a 15 cm/6 in cake tin. Cream together the Tomor and sugar, then beat in the eggs and vanilla essence. In a separate bowl, sift together the ground rice, baking powder and salt. Beat these dry ingredients into the egg, sugar and Tomor mixture. Add only a little water to obtain a firm but soft consistency; too much will cause the rice to sink in the middle during baking.

Turn the mixture into the greased cake tin and bake for 30–40 minutes, until golden brown. Do not open the oven door during baking.

Honey cake

See photograph, page 101

For a 15 cm/6 in diameter cake tin ★ W M E

150 ml/¼ pint runny honey
150 ml/¼ pint soya oil
½ sachet gelatine, dissolved in 150 ml/¼ pint hot water and left to cool to room temperature
225 g/8 oz buckwheat flour
5 tsp wheat-free baking powder (see page 95)

For the filling:
120 g/4 oz Tomor margarine
60 g/2 oz icing sugar
a little soya milk

Preheat the oven to 180°C/350°F/gas 4.

Grease a 15 cm/6 in diameter cake tin with Tomor and line the base and sides with foil. Beat together the honey, oil and the

---

Poached peaches with raspberry sauce (*left*, see page 112); Glazed pears with sultanas (*right*, see page 114)

gelatine solution. Sift the flour and baking powder together. Beat into the wet ingredients. Turn the mixture into the cake tin and bake for 40–45 minutes or until a skewer comes out clean when pushed into the centre.

Remove from the oven and leave to cool in the tin for a few minutes, then turn out on a wire tray. When the cake is quite cool, halve it. Make the cream filling by beating together the Tomor, sugar and enough milk to achieve a creamy consistency. Spread half the filling on the bottom half of the cake and press the top half firmly down on top. Cover with remaining filling. Decorate with seasonal fresh fruit.

Banana bake

For a 15 cm/6 in diameter cake tin W M

100 g/3½ oz ground rice
2 tsp wheat-free baking powder (see page 95)
1 pinch salt
½ tsp ground cinnamon
75 g/2½ oz muscovado sugar
30 g/1 oz Tomor margarine
50 g/1½ oz mixed sultanas and currants
1 large banana, mashed
1 egg

Preheat the oven to 190°C/375°F/gas 5.

Sift the ground rice and baking powder, salt and cinnamon together. Mix in the sugar. Add the chopped Tomor, together with the sultanas and currants and the banana. Mix well and then add the egg. Beat the mixture until smooth and well blended.

Grease a 15 cm/6 in diameter baking tin with Tomor. Pour the mixture into the tin and bake in the oven for 50 minutes.

After removing from the oven, leave the banana bake to stand for a few minutes, then turn out to cool on a wire tray.

Egg-free banana bake

For a 15 cm/6 in diameter cake tin W M E

100 g/3½ oz ground rice
2 tsp wheat-free baking powder (see page 95)
1 pinch salt
½ tsp ground cinnamon
75 g/2½ oz muscovado sugar
30 g/1 oz Tomor margarine, coarsely chopped
50 g/1½ oz mixed sultanas and currants
1 large mashed banana
½ sachet gelatine, dissolved in 90 ml/3 fl oz very hot water and left to cool to room temperature

Preheat the oven to 190°C/375°F/gas 5.

Sift together the rice, baking powder, salt, cinnamon and sugar. Add the chopped Tomor, and the dried fruit and banana. Mix well. Add the gelatine mixture. Beat until smooth.

Grease a 15 cm/6 in cake tin with Tomor. Pour the mixture into the tin and bake for 40–50 minutes. Remove from the oven and allow to stand in the tin for a few minutes. Turn on to a wire tray to cool completely.

Carrot cake

W M

Makes 24 slices

4 eggs
225 g/8 oz caster sugar
grated rind of 1 lemon
225 g/8 oz ground almonds
225 g/8 oz carrots, finely grated
1½ tbsp rice flour
1 tsp wheat-free baking powder (see page 95)

Preheat the oven to 180°C/350°F/gas 4.

Separate the eggs. Place the yolks, sugar and lemon rind in a bowl or in an electric blender and beat together well (about 5 minutes in the blender). Add the almonds and carrots to this mixture. Stir well. Sift the flour and baking powder together, then gradually fold them into the mixture. In another bowl, beat the egg whites until they are stiff, then fold them into the mixture.

Using Tomor, grease an oblong baking tray, 20 × 30 × 5 cm deep (8 × 12 × 2 in deep). Spread the mixture out in the tray and bake for 45 minutes. Leave to cool in the tray. Cut into slices when cool.

Note: The lemon can be omitted if not allowed.

Spiced biscuits

★ W M E

Makes 24 biscuits

85 g/3 oz buckwheat flour
85 g/3 oz rice flour
1 tbsp wheat-free baking powder (see page 95)
1 tsp ground ginger
½ tsp ground cinnamon
60 g/2 oz Tomor margarine
60 g/2 oz caster sugar
85 g/3 oz golden syrup, warmed

Preheat the oven to 200°C/400°F/gas 6.

Sift the buckwheat flour twice, discarding the tough black strands. Sift the sieved buckwheat flour with the rice flour, baking powder and spices twice. Rub in the margarine. Add the sugar and the syrup. Mix thoroughly.

Roll the mixture into balls and place them on a baking tray which has been greased with Tomor. Leave plenty of room between the balls to allow for spreading. Bake for 10–12 minutes.

Allow the biscuits to cool on the tray for a few minutes before transferring them to a wire cooling rack.

Almond biscuits

Makes 18–20 biscuits W M

120 g/4 oz rice flour
1½ tsp wheat-free baking powder (see page 95)
1 pinch salt
1 tsp mixed spice
60 ml/2 fl oz olive oil
60 g/2 oz soft brown sugar
60 g/2 oz caster sugar
1 egg, well beaten
¼ tsp almond essence
30 g/1 oz flaked almonds

Preheat the oven to 200°C/400°F/gas 6.

Sift the flour, baking powder, salt and spice together twice. Add the oil, sugars, egg and almond essence. Mix thoroughly.

Grease a baking tray with Tomor. Place teaspoons of the mixture on the tray, leaving plenty of space for spreading. Decorate with 2 flaked almonds per biscuit and bake for 10–12 minutes. Cool on a wire tray.

Coconut cookies

Makes 20 cookies ★ W M E

170 g/6 oz millet flour
1 tsp wheat-free baking powder (see page 95)
85 g/3 oz caster sugar
60 g/2 oz desiccated coconut
150 g/5 oz Tomor margarine

Preheat the oven to 160°C/325°F/gas 3.

Sift the flour and baking powder together into a mixing bowl. Add the sugar and coconut. Mix well. Rub in the margarine and knead well.

Dust a board and pin with millet flour. Roll out the mixture to 5 mm/¼ in thickness. Cut into rounds with a 4 cm/1½ in cutter.

Grease a baking tray with Tomor. Place the rounds on it and bake for approximately 15 minutes. Transfer to a wire tray to cool.

Orange biscuits

Makes 24 biscuits W M

225 g/8 oz rice flour
1 tsp wheat-free baking powder (see page 95)
120 g/4 oz Tomor margarine
1 egg, well beaten
juice of ½ an orange
rind of ½ an orange, finely grated

Preheat the oven to 160°C/325°F/gas 3.

Sift the flour and baking powder together twice. Rub in the margarine. Add the egg, orange juice and rind. Mix thoroughly.

Dust a board and pin with rice flour. Roll out the mixture to 5 mm/¼ in thickness. Cut into rounds. Grease a baking tray with Tomor and put the rounds on it, leaving room for spreading. Bake for approximately 15 minutes.

Transfer to a wire tray to cool.

Ginger biscuits

See photograph, page 101

Makes about 18/20 biscuits ★ W M E

200 g/7 oz ground rice
2 tsp wheat-free baking powder (see page 95)
2 tsp ground ginger
75 g/2½ oz muscovado sugar
75 g/2½ oz Tomor margarine
a little water
a little rice flour

Preheat the oven to 190°C/375°F/gas 5.

Sift together the baking powder, ginger and sugar. Add the ground rice. Chop the Tomor into pieces, add it to the dry ingredients and rub it in evenly and thoroughly to achieve a crumbly consistency. When the ingredients are well mixed, add just enough water to obtain a soft dough.

Dust a board and rolling pin with rice flour. Grease a large baking tray with Tomor. Roll out the dough to a thickness of 1.25 cm /½ in. Cut into interesting shapes. Carefully place the dough shapes on the baking tray and bake in the oven for 20–25 minutes. Remove from the oven and leave to cool on a wire tray.

Coconut rice biscuits

Makes about 18/20 biscuits W M

75 g/2½ oz Tomor margarine
75 g/2½ oz muscovado sugar
1 small egg
200 g/7 oz ground rice
1 tsp wheat-free baking powder (see page 95)
75 g/2½ oz desiccated coconut

Preheat the oven to 190°C/375°F/gas 5.

Cream together the Tomor and sugar. Beat in the egg. In a separate bowl, sift together the ground rice, and baking powder, then mix in the coconut. Add these ingredients to the Tomor/sugar/egg mixture and beat until smooth. Turn out onto a surface which has been lightly dusted with rice flour and knead until smooth. Roll the dough out to a thickness of 1.25 cm/½ in. Cut into rounds with a biscuit cutter.

Grease a large baking tray with Tomor and carefully transfer the dough shapes on to it. Bake in the middle of the oven for 15–20 minutes. Leave the biscuits to cool on a wire tray.

Elevenses

Makes 8 fingers ★ W M E

50 g/1½ oz carob flour
75 g/2½ oz ground rice
50 g/1½ oz granulated sugar
1 tsp wheat-free baking powder (see page 95)
50 g/1½ oz Tomor margarine
½ sachet gelatine, dissolved in 120 ml/4 fl oz hot water and left to cool to room temperature

Preheat the oven to 180°C/350°F/gas 4.

Grease a large baking tray with Tomor. Sift together the dry ingredients. Chop the Tomor into pieces and rub it in, evenly and thoroughly. Stir in the gelatine solution and mix to make a firm dough.

Dust the rolling pin and a board with carob flour and roll out the dough until it is 1.25 cm/½ in thick. Cut it into 8 fingers and transfer them to the baking tray, using a palette knife.

Bake for 10 minutes then cool on a wire tray.

Parkin

For an 18 × 23 cm/7 × 9 in cake tin ★ W M E

225 g/8 oz millet flour
1 tsp bicarbonate of soda
2 tsp ground ginger
225 g/8 oz millet flakes
120 g/4 oz Tomor margarine
120 ml/4 fl oz molasses
120 ml/4 fl oz golden syrup
2 tbsp runny honey
1 tbsp soft brown sugar
180 ml/6 fl oz milk substitute

Preheat the oven to 180°C/350°F/gas 4.

Sift the flour, bicarbonate of soda and ginger into a bowl. Stir in the millet flakes. Place the Tomor, molasses, golden syrup, honey and sugar in a pan. Gently heat the pan until all the ingredients are melted. Remove from the heat and beat into the flour mixture with the milk substitute.

Grease a 18 × 23 cm/7 × 9 in cake tin with Tomor. Pour the mixture into the tin and bake for 45–50 minutes until it is firm to the touch. Leave to cool in the tin for 15 minutes, then turn out on a cooling rack.

Millet flake digestives

Makes 25–30 biscuits W M

120 g/4 oz potato flour
⅛ tsp salt
85 g/3 oz Tomor margarine
120 g/4 oz millet flakes
30 g/1 oz brown sugar
1 egg

Preheat the oven to 180°C/350°F/gas 4.

Sift the flour and salt together. Rub the margarine into the flour. Stir in the millet flakes and brown sugar. Add the egg and mix well until a firm dough is formed.

Dust a board and pin with potato flour and roll out the dough to 5 mm/¼ in thick. Cut into rounds with a 5 cm/2 in cutter. Prick each biscuit with a fork and place on a baking tray which has been greased with Tomor. Bake for 15–20 minutes until the biscuits are golden brown. Leave in the tray to cool.

Date and millet squares

Makes 16 squares ★ W M E

225 g/8 oz dates, chopped
120 ml/4 fl oz apple juice
120 g/4 oz Tomor margarine
170 g/6 oz soft brown sugar
120 g/4 oz rice or millet flour
170 g/6 oz millet flakes

Preheat the oven to 180°C/350°F/gas 4.

Put the dates in a pan, pour in the apple juice and cook over a gentle heat until the mixture is soft and pulpy (about 5 minutes). Chop the margarine into small pieces. Place the sugar, rice or millet flour and millet flakes in a bowl, add the chopped margarine and mix until all the ingredients are combined.

Grease a 18 × 23 cm/7 × 9 in baking tin. Divide the millet mixture in half. Press half the mixture firmly into the bottom of the tin and spread the date mixture over the top. Cover with the remaining millet mixture and press down firmly.

Bake for 35–40 minutes. Allow to cool in the tin. Cut into squares when cold.

FRUIT AND PUDDINGS

Banana cream

Serves 4

W M E

4 medium bananas
1 tbsp lemon juice
400 ml/14 fl oz goat's or ewe's yoghurt
1 tsp honey

Place all ingredients in the blender and liquidize until creamy. Chill well before serving.

Italian baked peaches

Serves 6

W M E

6 large peaches
120 g/4 oz ground almonds
60 g/2 oz soft brown sugar
60 ml/2 fl oz apple juice

Preheat the oven to 220°C/425°F/gas 7.

Plunge the peaches into boiling water for a few minutes. Remove and peel them. Cut in half and remove the stones.

Mix together the ground almonds and the brown sugar. Add just enough apple juice to moisten the mixture – approximately 1 tbsp. Stuff the peaches with the mixture, filling the holes left by the stones. Press the halves back together.

Place the peaches in an ovenproof dish. Pour over the remaining apple juice. Cover the dish and bake in the oven for 30–40 minutes, until the peaches are tender.

Poached peaches with raspberry sauce

See photograph, page 104

Serves 4

★ W M E

4 large peaches
150 ml/¼ pint water
½ tsp vanilla essence
120 g/4 oz sugar

For the sauce:
150 g/5 oz raspberries
50 g/1½ oz icing sugar
1½ tsp grape juice

Plunge the peaches into boiling water for a few minutes. Remove and peel them. Place the 150 ml/¼ pint water in a pan, add the vanilla essence and sugar. Poach the peaches in this syrup until tender – about 30 minutes, depending on size. Remove the peaches and leave them to cool.

Make the sauce by placing the raspberries in a dish. Sprinkle the sugar over the raspberries. Spoon the grape juice over the top and leave to marinate for at least 1 hour. Place the mixture in a blender and liquidize to a purée. Sieve and chill.

Put the peaches into individual dishes, pour some sauce on each one and serve.

Savoleyres special

Makes 900 ml/1½ pints ★ W M E

450 g/1 lb fresh apricots
600 ml/1 pint water
170 g/6 oz sugar
4 tbsp apple juice

Place the apricots and the water in a pan. Add the sugar and bring to the boil. Simmer gently until the apricots are soft. Leave to cool, then remove the skins and the stones.

Place the apricots and the syrup in the blender, add the apple juice and liquidize to a purée.

Green fruit mousse

Serves 4–6 ★ W M E

450 g/1 lb seedless green grapes
225 g/8 oz gooseberries, topped and tailed
170 g/6 oz caster sugar
75 ml/2½ fl oz apple juice
15 g/½ oz sachet powdered gelatine
150 ml/¼ pint goat's yoghurt
1 kiwi fruit for decoration

Place the grapes, gooseberries, sugar and apple juice in a pan. Bring to the boil and simmer for 20 minutes. Leave to cool, then liquidize. Pass the mixture through a sieve to obtain as much juice as possible. Dissolve the gelatine in a little hot water and add this to the juice. Stir in the yoghurt. Pour into individual glass dishes and leave to set.

Just before serving, peel and slice the kiwi fruit and use to decorate the mousse.

Glazed pears with sultanas ★ W M E

Serves 2

See photograph, page 104

2 ripe pears
60 ml/2 fl oz water
30 g/1 oz sultanas
1 tbsp honey
20 g/½ oz brown sugar

Preheat the oven to 190°C/375°F/gas 5.

Peel the pears, leaving on the stalks. Core from the base. Divide the sultanas between the two pears and use to stuff the cavities. Place in a shallow ovenproof dish with the water and the sultanas. Spread the honey evenly over the pears and sprinkle the brown sugar on top. Place in the oven and cook for 30 minutes.

Melon shells filled with fruit ★ W M E A

Serves 6

1 melon
4 peaches, sliced
450 g/1 lb red grapes, cut in half and seeded

Cut the melon in half lengthways. Remove the seeds. Being careful not to damage the skin, scoop out the melon flesh and cut it into cubes. Set the skins aside. Put the melon cubes into a bowl and add the sliced peaches and the prepared grapes. Mix the fruit carefully.

Fill the melon halves with the fruit mixture, dividing it equally between the two. Chill for 30 minutes in the refrigerator before serving.

Note: Any combination of fruit fillings can be used, depending on the season. For example, strawberries, raspberries, nectarines, kiwi fruit.

Apple brulée ★ W M E

Serves 1

1 small baking apple
sugar
a little water
4 tbsp goat's milk yoghurt
1 tbsp demerara sugar

Stew the apple with as little water as possible, and sugar to taste. Allow to cool.

Place the apple in an individual ovenproof dish. Top with the yoghurt and then the demerara sugar. Place under a hot grill until the sugar melts and bubbles. Serve immediately.

Fancy fruit

★ W M E A

Serves 2

1 kiwi fruit
2 peaches or nectarines
1 banana
1 mango

Wash and skin the kiwi fruit. Slice it crossways, so the lovely radiating pattern is revealed. Arrange the discs around the edge of a dinner plate.

Stone the peaches/nectarines and cut them into 'new moons'. Arrange these between the kiwi discs. Peel and chop the banana and arrange the banana discs inside the ring of kiwi and peach/nectarine slices. Finally, halve the mango, scoop out balls of the flesh (with a melon-baller if you have one) and pile the mango flesh in the middle of the plate.

Delicious served chilled.

A taste of summer

★ W M E

Serves 3

400 g/14 oz rhubarb
200 g/7 oz blackcurrants
1 nectarine
1 tbsp granulated sugar
300 ml/½ pint water

Wash and chop the rhubarb. Prepare the blackcurrants. Stone and coarsely chop the nectarine. Layer the three fruits in a heatproof bowl, sprinkling the layers with sugar as you go. Cover the bowl with a double layer of greaseproof paper and fasten securely.

Place the trivet and water in the pressure cooker. Lower the bowl in. Cook at high pressure for 7 minutes, then reduce the pressure quickly by running cold water over the pressure cooker in the sink. Remove the bowl and allow the fruit to cool at room temperature.

Note: This method of cooking preserves flavours well and allows the fruit to retain its shape.

Cinnamon rhubarb

★ W M E

Serves 3

300 g/11 oz rhubarb
4 tbsp water
1 pinch cinnamon
50–60 g/1½–2 oz granulated or muscovado sugar

Wash and chop the rhubarb. Place it in a pan with the water, cinnamon and sugar. Gently stew the mixture until the rhubarb is tender.

Note: Muscovado sugar gives a delicious rich flavour.

Baked apples

★ W M E

Serves 2

2 large cooking apples
2 tbsp demerara sugar
2 pinches ground cinnamon
2 pinches freshly ground nutmeg
2 tbsp currants
2 cloves

Preheat the oven to 190°C/375°F/gas 5.

Core the apples, being careful not to damage the outsides. In a bowl, combine the sugar, cinnamon and nutmeg.

Stand the apples in a suitable size baking tray. Pack the hollow centres with alternate layers of dried fruit and the sugar/spice mixture. Remember to include 1 clove in each apple – but do warn people to be careful not to swallow them!

Bake for about 20 minutes and serve with coconut sauce (see page 93).

Blackcurrant and tofu whip

See photograph, page 103

★ W M E A

Serves 4–6

450 g/1 lb ripe blackcurrants
a little water
sugar to taste (omit if following the arthritis exclusion diet)
280 g/10 oz tofu

Place the blackcurrants in a pan with the water and sugar to taste. Bring to the boil and stew until the blackcurrants are tender. Leave to cool. Place in the blender with the tofu and liquidize until smooth. Chill well before serving.

Note: Other fruits such as blackberries or gooseberries can be substituted for the blackcurrants in this recipe.

Carob ice cream

See photograph, page 103

Serves 4–6

★ W M E

60 g/2 oz runny honey
500 ml/18 fl oz soya milk
4 tbsp sunflower oil
¼ tsp salt
60 g/2 oz carob powder

Place all ingredients in the blender and liquidize until smooth. Place in a suitable container and freeze for approximately 3 hours, until the mixture begins to set. Beat with a fork, then return to the freezer to firm up for at least 1 hour.

Transfer to the refrigerator 30 minutes before serving, to allow the ice cream to soften.

Note: This ice cream can be made with other flavourings besides carob powder, such as puréed fruit.

Millet and hazelnut ice

W M

Serves 6–8

See photograph, page 103

85 g/3 oz millet flakes
60 g/2 oz chopped hazelnuts
170 g/6 oz muscovado sugar
3 egg whites
300 ml/½ pint goat's or ewe's yoghurt

Place the millet flakes, chopped hazelnuts and 60 g/2 oz of the sugar in a bowl. Mix together. Spread out on a baking sheet and place under a preheated grill for a few minutes until browned, stirring occasionally. Leave to cool.

Whisk the egg whites until stiff. Gradually whisk in the remaining sugar. Carefully fold in the yoghurt and toasted millet/hazelnut mixture. Turn into a freezerproof container, cover, seal and freeze for 4–5 hours, until firm.

Transfer to the refrigerator 30 minutes before serving, to allow the ice cream to soften.

Rice and carob pudding

W M E

Serves 2

300 ml/½ pint milk substitute
2 tbsp ground rice
1 tbsp demerara sugar
2 tbsp desiccated coconut
3 tbsp ground almonds
2 tsp carob flour
a little extra desiccated coconut

Pour the milk substitute into a pan and heat to boiling point. Sprinkle the ground rice and demerara sugar into the milk and cook gently, stirring continuously, until the pudding thickens (about 4 minutes). Stir in the coconut, ground almonds and carob flour. Mix well.

Serve hot or cold in individual dishes, sprinkling each portion with a little coconut before serving.

Christmas pudding

W M

Makes 1 large or 2 medium puddings

170 g/6 oz Tomor margarine
225 g/8 oz soft brown sugar
3 eggs
675 g/1½ lb mixed dried fruit
60 g/2 oz flaked almonds
1 small dessert apple, cored, peeled and grated
finely grated rind of ½ an orange
60 g/2 oz potato flour
60 g/2 oz rice flour or ground rice
¼ tsp freshly grated nutmeg
½ tsp mixed spice
2–3 tbsp brandy

Cream the Tomor and sugar together. In a separate bowl beat the eggs, then add them to the Tomor/sugar a little at a time, beating continuously. Add the dried fruit, almonds, grated apple and orange rind and mix well. Sift together the flours, nutmeg and mixed spice and add to the mixture. Stir in the brandy.

Place the mixture in pudding basins which have been greased with Tomor, cover with greaseproof paper or foil. Steam for 3 hours.

Note: The puddings will not keep as long as ordinary Christmas puddings. It is best to freeze them for storage.

Cambridge dariole

W M

For a 19 cm/7½ in flan tin

2 eggs
2 egg whites (eg, those left from making the pâte sucrée)
300 ml/½ pint soya milk
50 g/1½ oz sugar
1 recipe pâte sucrée, baked blind (see page 99)

Preheat the oven to 180°C/350°F/gas 4.

Beat together the eggs, egg whites, the soya milk and the sugar. Then strain this custard mixture into the prepared pâte sucrée case. Bake for 30–40 minutes, until the custard is just set. Serve cold.

To observe Cambridge tradition, the dariole should be served with redcurrant jelly. (Don't forget to check the label.)

Note: Strictly speaking, darioles should be made in small tins. You could make 3 or 4 with the quantities given in this recipe, but it is easier to make a large one with the wheat-free pâte sucrée.

Autumn tart

★ W M E

For a 23 cm/9 in flan tin

60 g/2 oz Tomor margarine
2 pinches ground ginger
210 g/7½ oz crushed coconut rice biscuits (see page 109)
650 g/1 lb 7 oz apples (a mixture of cooking apples and a couple of dessert apples)
120 ml/4 fl oz water
60 g/2 oz muscovado sugar
3 cloves
1 pinch cinnamon
60 g/2 oz sultanas
1 sachet gelatine

Melt the Tomor in a pan. Stir in the ginger, then stir in the crushed biscuits. Mix well. Grease a 23 cm/9 in flan tin or dish with Tomor. Press the biscuit mixture into the bottom of the tin. Place in the refrigerator to chill.

Peel, core and chop the apples. Place them in a pan with the water, sugar, spices and sultanas and bring to the boil. Turn down the heat and stew the mixture slowly, stirring gently so that the apple does not break up. Drain the apples, reserving the cooking liquid.

Make the cooking liquid up to 160 ml/6 fl oz with hot water. Briskly stir in the gelatine powder. Allow both the gelatine and the apples to cool to room temperature. Remove the cloves from the apples and combine the apples with the gelatine. Leave until the gelatine has nearly set. Turn on to the biscuit base in the flan dish. Allow to set firmly before serving.

Note: Other allergy-free biscuits can be substituted for the coconut rice biscuits in this recipe, in which case you may prefer to exclude the ginger.

APPENDIX: FOOD LABELLING

The following serial numbers may be used on food labels in the UK as alternatives to the names of additives.

Serial number	*Name of additive*
E 100	curcumin
E101	riboflavin or lactoflavin
E102	tartrazine
E104	quinoline yellow
E110	sunset yellow FCF or orange yellow S
E120	cochineal or carminic acid
E122	carmoisine or azorubine
E123	amaranth
E124	ponceau 4R or cochineal red A
E127	erythrosine BS
E131	patent blue V
E132	indigo carmine or indigotine
E140	chlorophyll
E141	copper complexes of chlorophyll and chlorophyllins
E142	green S or acid brilliant green BS or lissamine green
E150	caramel
E151	black PN or brilliant black BN
E153	carbon black or vegetable carbon
E160(a)	alpha-carotene, beta-carotene, gamma-carotene
E160(b)	annatto, bixin, norbixin
E160(c)	capsanthin or capsorubin
E160(d)	lycopene
E160(e)	beta-apo-8′-carotenal (C30)
E160(f)	ethyl ester of beta-apo-8′-carotenoic acid (C30)
E161(a)	flavoxanthin
E161(b)	lutein
E161(c)	cryptoxanthin
E161(d)	rubixanthin
E161(e)	violaxanthin
E161(f)	rhodoxanthin
E161(g)	canthaxanthin
E162	beetroot red or betanin
E163	anthocyanins
E170	calcium carbonate
E171	titanium dioxide
E172	iron oxide and hydroxides
E173	aluminium
E174	silver
E175	gold
E180	pigment rubine or lithol rubine BK
E200	sorbic acid
E201	sodium sorbate
E202	potassium sorbate
E203	calcium sorbate
E210	benzoic acid
E211	sodium benzoate

E212	potassium benzoate
E213	calcium benzoate
E214	ethyl 4-hydroxybenzoate
E215	ethyl 4-hydroxybenzoate sodium salt
E216	propyl 4-hydroxybenzoate
E217	propyl 4-hydroxybenzoate sodium salt
E218	methyl 4-hydroxybenzoate
E219	methyl 4-hydroxybenzoate sodium salt
E220	sulphur dioxide
E221	sodium sulphite
E222	sodium hydrogen sulphite
E223	sodium metabisulphite
E224	potassium metabisulphite
E226	calcium sulphite
E227	calcium hydrogen sulphite
E230	biphenyl or diphenyl
E231	2-hydroxybiphenyl
E232	sodium biphenyl-2-yl-oxide
E233	2-(thiazol-4-yl) benzimidazole
E236	formic acid
E237	sodium formate
E238	calcium formate
E239	hexamine
E249	potassium nitrite
E250	sodium nitrite
E251	sodium nitrate
E252	potassium nitrate
E260	acetic acid
E261	potassium acetate
E262	sodium hydrogen diacetate
E263	calcium acetate
E270	lactic acid
E280	propionic acid
E281	sodium propionate
E282	calcium propionate
E283	potassium propionate
E290	carbon dioxide
E300	L-ascorbic acid
E301	sodium-L-ascorbate
E302	calcium-L-ascorbate
E304	6-O-palmitoyl-L-ascorbic acid
E306	extracts of natural origin rich in tocopherols
E307	synthetic alpha-tocopherol
E308	synthetic gamma-tocopherol
E309	synthetic delta-tocopherol
E310	propyl gallate
E311	octyl gallate
E312	dodecyl gallate
E320	butylated hydroxyanisole
E321	butylated hydroxytoluene
E322	lecithins
E325	sodium lactate
E326	potassium lactate
E327	calcium lactate

E330	citric acid
E331	sodium dihydrogen citrate
E331	disodium citrate
E331	trisodium citrate
E332	potassium dihydrogen citrate
E332	tripotassium citrate
E333	calcium citrate
E333	dicalcium citrate
E333	tricalcium citrate
E334	tartaric acid
E335	sodium tartrate
E336	potassium tartrate
E336	potassium hydrogen tartrate
E337	potassium sodium tartrate
E338	orthophosphoric acid
E339(a)	sodium dihydrogen orthophosphate
E339(b)	disodium hydrogen orthophosphate
E339(c)	trisodium orthophosphate
E340(a)	potassium dihydrogen orthophosphate
E340(b)	dipotassium hydrogen orthophosphate
E340(c)	tripotassium orthophosphate
E341(a)	calcium tetrahydrogen diorthophosphate
E341(b)	calcium hydrogen orthophosphate
E341(c)	tricalcium diorthophosphate
E400	alginic acid
E401	sodium alginate
E402	potassium alginate
E403	ammonium alginate
E404	calcium alginate
E405	propane-1, 2-diol alginate
E406	agar
E407	carrageenan
E410	locust bean gum
E412	guar gum
E413	tragacanth
E414	acacia or gum arabic
E415	xanthan gum
E420(i)	sorbitol
E420(ii)	sorbitol syrup
E421	mannitol
E422	glycerol
E440(a)	pectin
E440(b)	pectin, amidated
E450(a)	disodium dihydrogen diphosphate
E450(a)	tetrasodium diphosphate
E450(a)	tetrapotassium diphosphate
E450(a)	trisodium diphosphate
E450(b)	pentasodium triphosphate
E450(b)	pentapotassium triphosphate
E450(c)	sodium polyphosphate
E450(c)	potassium polyphosphates
E460(i)	microcrystalline cellulose
E460(ii)	powdered cellulose
E461	methylcellulose

E463	hydroxypropylcellulose
E464	hydroxypropylmethylcellulose
E465	ethylmethylcellulose
E466	carboxymethylcellulose, sodium salt
E470	sodium potassium and calcium salts of fatty acids
E471	mono- and di-glycerides of fatty acids
E472(a)	acetic acid esters of mono- and di-glycerides of fatty acids
E472(b)	lactic acid esters of mono- and di-glycerides of fatty acids
E472(c)	citric acid esters of mono- and di-glycerides of fatty acids
E472(d)	tartaric acid esters of mono- and di-glycerides of fatty acids
E472(e)	diacetyltartaric acid esters of mono- and di-glycerides of fatty acids
E473	sucrose esters of fatty acids
E474	sucroglycerides
E475	polyglycerol esters of fatty acids
E477	propane-1, 2-diol esters of fatty acids
E481	sodium stearoyl-2-lactylate
E482	calcium stearoyl-2-lactylate
E483	stearyl tartrate

Since they have hardly ever produced symptoms, substances denoted by the following E numbers are permitted on the first stage of the exclusion diet.

E100
E101
E120
E140
E150
E153
E160a
E160b
E160c
E160d
E161a
E161b
E161c
E161d
E161e
E161f
E161g
E162
E170
E172
E290
E296
E297
E300
E301
E302
E306
E307
E308
E309
E322
E336
E363
E375
E400
E404
E406
E407
E410
E412
E413
E414
E415
E416
E420(i)
E420(ii)
E421
E422
E440(a)
E440(b)
E460(i)
E460(ii)
E466
E500
E501
E504
E508
E509
E515
E516
E518
E529
E530
E542
E559
E901
E903
E904

ACKNOWLEDGMENTS

The authors are particularly grateful to Alison Wilson for typing the manuscript.

1986

EW
VAJ
JH

The publishers are grateful to the following for their help in preparation of this book: the photographs were taken by Ray Moller, assisted by Liz Gedney; art direction was by Valerie Wright, styling by Penny Markham and food preparation by Lisa Collard.

INDEX

Page numbers in *italic* refer to the illustrations